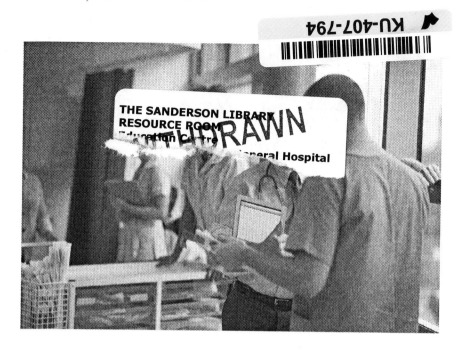

Clinical Leadership:

A Practical Guide for Tutors, Trainees & Practitioners

Professor Peter Spurgeon, Paul W Long, Jane Powell, Professor Mary Lovegrove

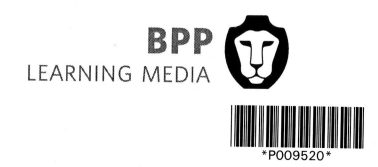

BPP
LEARNING MEDIA

First edition June 2015

ISBN 9781 4727 2783 1
eISBN 9781 4727 3928 5

British Library Cataloguing-in-Publication Data
A catalogue record for this book is available from
the British Library

Published by
BPP Learning Media Ltd
BPP House, Aldine Place
London W12 8AA

www.bpp.com/health

Printed in the United Kingdom by RICOH UK
Limited

Unit 2
Wells Place
Merstham
RH1 3LG

Your learning materials, published by BPP
Learning Media Ltd, are printed on paper
sourced from sustainable, managed forests.

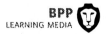

About the publisher

BPP Learning Media is dedicated to supporting aspiring professionals with top quality learning material. BPP Learning Media's commitment to success is shown by our record of quality, innovation and market leadership in paper-based and e-learning materials. BPP Learning Media's study materials are written by professionally-qualified specialists who know from personal experience the importance of top quality materials for success.

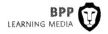

Contents

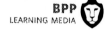

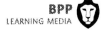

Contents

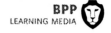

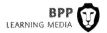

About the authors

Professor P Spurgeon

Professor Peter Spurgeon is a previous Director of the Health Services Management Centre, University of Birmingham and established the Institute of Clinical Leadership at the Medical School, Warwick University. He led the national project that developed the Medical Leadership Competency Framework (MLCF) which was endorsed by the General Medical Council and subsequently adapted for all clinical professionals as the Clinical Leadership Competency Framework (CLCF). He leads the work nationally and internationally on medical engagement and its link to organisational performance. Currently he is also working on a new, proactive risk based approach to improving patient safety and also measuring organisational safety culture.

Paul W. Long

Is the author of many high profile reports, articles and academic papers, on systems approaches to improving the quality of healthcare. Paul lived in the United Kingdom for a number of years where he led research to test the applicability of generic leadership competences across all of the clinical professions. Paul's work was recognised when, in July 2011, the then Secretary of State for Health launched the new NHS Leadership Framework and companion Clinical Leadership Competency Framework. Now living in Australia and running a busy management consultancy practice, Paul is a graduate of Harvard University Kennedy School, and a Visiting Fellow of the Faculty of Medicine and Health Sciences, Australian Institute for Health Innovation, Macquarie University.

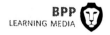

Jane Powell

Jane is a registered nurse with over 28 years' experience in healthcare. Jane has spent most of her clinical time in cardiology and has held senior management posts at local and regional level, becoming West Midlands Regional Coordinator for the implementation of the Coronary Heart Disease National Service Framework and representing the West Midlands on national committees at the Department of Health. She has been an advisor to the Commission for Health Improvement now the Care Quality Commission. Also Jane has worked in academia as Director for Business Development and Innovation and as an independent healthcare consultant working with the World Health Organisation. Jane is currently the Clinical Operations Manager for a national wound care company.

Prof Mary Lovegrove, OBE

Mary Lovegrove is a Diagnostic Radiographer by profession. In 2012 she was awarded an OBE for her work supporting Allied Health Professions. She currently has a portfolio career partly as International Lead for the School of Health and Social Care based at the London South Bank University and as Director of Allied Health Solutions. She holds a personal chair in Education and Development of Allied Health Professionals with particular interests in clinical leadership, service transformation and workforce development. Mary's contribution has gone beyond her own profession to being a strong advocate of all Allied Health professionals. This has led her to make significant contributions to the education and development of the clinical professional workforce. Mary also has long-standing international interests overseas particularly in the Far East (Hong Kong, Malaysia and Singapore) where she continues to have an education advisory role.

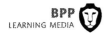

Case study contributors

Alexia Zeniou-Lad , BSc (Hons) Nursing (Adult), Staff Nurse, Critical Care

James Taylor, Paramedic

Mr Kit Tse, Pharmacist, Tse Consulting Limited

Dr Keith Ison, Head of Medical Physics, Guy's and St Thomas' NHS Foundation Trust

Philippa Bridgeman, Clinical Nurse, Specialist Limb Reconstruction, University Hospital Birmingham NHS Foundation Trust

Paula Clarke, Consultant Midwife Birmingham Women's Hospital NHS Foundation Trust

Derek Farrell, Senior Lecturer, Institute Health Studies, University of Worcester

Penny Lewis, Occupational Therapist and Independent Consultant, Tony and Penny Lewis Associates

Prof Rebecca Jester, Head of Dept, Adult Nursing and Midwifery Studies, London South Bank University

Naomi Parsons, Student Midwife, Faculty of Health and Social Care of the University of Chester

Angela Penswick, Matron Lister Unit and James Ward, North West London Hospitals NHS Trust

Julie Foley, Midwife Supervisor, Imperial College Healthcare NHS Trust

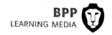

Acknowledgements

Peter Spurgeon and Paul W Long

We would like to acknowledge and thank our colleagues on the Clinical Leadership Competency Framework Project team – Tracy Lonetto, Sue Balderson, Kate Gosney, John Clark; and later Sue Mortlock, Sabhia Sheikh together with Pippa Cronk who worked with us on the NHS Leadership Framework – for making it a thoroughly enjoyable and satisfying experience. We would also like to thank our co-authors Jane Powell and Mary Lovegrove for their contacts and insight into clinical practice. Finally thanks also to Emma Darbey for so helpfully collating the material.

Paul W Long

On a personal note I'd like to add that I especially enjoy working with clinicians or other frontline staff. I have never met a clinician that didn't want to do better. They are busy, hardworking and often, hard pressed. Their time is precious so I feel privileged when they offer me some of their time.

I hope this text is helpful to them, and in some way better enables them to understand leadership and how it can make a difference to their practise and their patients.

I'd like to thank Peter for asking me to collaborate with him on this book and to especially thank Jenni Leigh from whom I learned a lot and owe a great deal for the friendship, wise counsel and stimulating collaboration over the past 14 years.

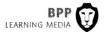

Foreword

I am pleased to provide the foreword for this important text which will be of enormous value to everyone involved in healthcare. At the time of writing, health services in the United Kingdom are under enormous scrutiny from a wide range of organisations and stakeholders. In the build up to the General Election the health service was one of the major battlegrounds and is likely to remain so for the foreseeable future following the General Election.

There is a crisis of confidence amongst many of the current leaders in healthcare and in the supply line of those who traditionally may have been expected to have progressed into leadership roles. This is amply demonstrated by the number of vacant Chief Executive posts for NHS Trusts and the number of vacancies for Director of Nursing or Finance.

Increasingly, many individuals from a clinical background are questioning whether it is worth undertaking the highly challenging and complex role of leadership in a climate that at times can be very unforgiving – not to mention misunderstood by politicians and the media. When getting underneath the hyperbole that surrounds discussion on health services, there are some emerging trends that are a source of encouragement.

The first is the trend to ensure that people from a clinical background are taking more of a leadership role both in the operational and strategic aspects of health services management. We are seeing an erosion of the traditional parallel lines between managers and clinicians. The agenda is the same, clinical work and patient care. Managers, clinicians and those in leadership roles should be there to help drive, develop and enhance the effectiveness of the respective organisations.

Change is needed to ensure that health needs are met – those health needs will include many people living longer, but not necessarily in good health. The complex and long term conditions which the health and social care services will need to deal with will need creative thinking and changes to the way services are delivered.

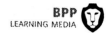

This text moves away from the traditional concept of leaders being strong, powerful and charismatic individuals and enhances the concept of shared leadership applicable to all engaged in clinical practice. It also emphasises the need to ensure that students, irrespective of their discipline, need to understand at a very early stage the critical elements required for good leadership and optimum organisational performance.

Hitherto, leadership and a broader awareness of organisational needs have tended to be something that has been an addendum or has been left to individuals who may have a particular interest in the subject. I would recommend that this text should be widely used in undergraduate and post graduate settings. It should also be used by those who are currently in leadership roles and would do well to adopt the clinical leadership competencies framework and the associated ideas and concepts that emerge from this.

I thoroughly recommend this book that I believe will become essential reading for all of those involved in health service leadership.

Peter Carter, OBE,
Chief Executive, Royal College of Nursing,
PhD, RMN & RGN.

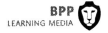

Chapter 1
Introduction

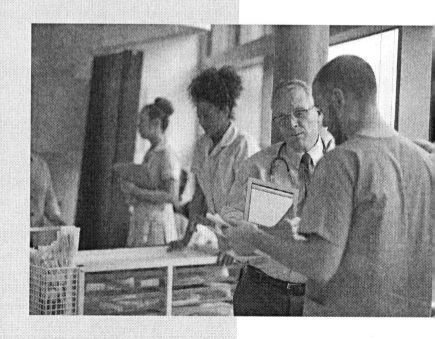

Introduction

Chapter overview

This chapter provides:

- An outline of the origins and background to the widespread demand for effective clinical leadership.

- A Framework for using this book, from early chapters which offer a conceptual background to those later chapters offering practical learning opportunities within meaningful patient contexts.

There is great interest in the process of leadership across all sectors in the UK, and in many other countries around the world. The literature is vast and in many instances overwhelming and confusing for the practitioner. No single agreed definition of leadership exists and hence authors will often proceed to talk about leadership and make the assumption that either the reader shares their particular understanding of the concept or that leadership is such an all-encompassing term that precise definition is not needed.

The model of leadership adopted can actually make quite a significant difference especially to the way in which training and development in leadership is approached. The traditional assumption of seeking a powerful, charismatic figure to be the leader tends to focus on personal qualities existing within the individual and therefore emphasises the notion that these qualities are inherent or in-built in certain special individuals. This is a slightly dated approach and undermined somewhat by the failure of much research activity to locate consistently just what these characteristics or traits are. It is also a bit dispiriting if you feel on reflection that you really do not possess some of these characteristics – implying that training is probably futile.

A more recent and modern conception is of leadership as a set of behaviours that can be learned to a lesser or greater degree by most people. They can then be applied and produced in a variety of different contexts. This is a more encouraging model offering some development potential to all to make a leadership contribution. This is very much the underlying approach of this text. However, it is not our intention to engage in a long winded debate about the merits, or otherwise, of various approaches. The emphasis

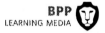

here is much more on practice and how clinical leadership has become such an important and central component of change and improvement in the health service.

The emergence and value of clinical leadership

The challenges facing the health system, in the UK and globally, are well rehearsed. Briefly the major pressures on Western health systems can be outlined as:

- New patterns of disease, with emphasis on chronic and multiple conditions.
- New techniques, technology and drugs placing a financial burden upon the total health budget.
- Increased expectations from patients and carers.
- An aging population with increasingly complex conditions exacerbated by diverse cultural needs.

Alongside this virtually all health systems are also having to tackle financial constraints with the UK system under pressure to save an unprecedented (worldwide) fifth of its total budget over four years. There is a strongly advocated view that the size of this challenge cannot be achieved without a strengthened and positively committed clinical leadership.

An interesting question posed by some (Edmonstone, 2009) is whether leadership – as widely advocated even if unspecified – is the same as clinical leadership. It might be argued that clinical leadership is just a description of any individual in a clinical role who exercises leadership, others suggest that it is leadership by clinicians for clinicians. The latter would seem a dangerously narrow formulation, almost by definition excluding other areas of management or leadership activity. This is not the concept of clinical leadership advanced here; rather we are discussing the skills of leadership directed by a person (clinician or not) to an area of activity that might secure improved patient care. Such leadership enactment would almost inevitably impact upon individuals other than clinicians alone. It is also a notion of leadership compatible with this simple, working definition 'Leadership is a process of influence whereby those subject to it are inspired, motivated or

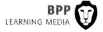

become willing to undertake the tasks necessary to achieve an agreed goal' (Spurgeon & Klaber, 2011).

Rather than seeking a potentially spurious definition of clinical leadership that separates it from other forms of leadership it might be more fruitful to consider the functions and contribution sought from clinical leadership (Storey & Holti, 2012). They suggest the key contributions as follows:

- To bring on board their professional colleagues.

- To utilise the unique clinical expertise to ensure that plans for change are feasible, are safe and will benefit patients.

- To provide external reassurance to patients and the public that they have the support of clinical professionals.

- To ensure the move to more integrated care builds upon the good practice of multi-professional teams.

This last point is especially important in the context of this text. Previous work by the NHS Institute for Innovation and Improvement and the Academy of Medical Royal Colleges sought to foster medical leadership and in the process devised the Medical Leadership Competency Framework (MLCF). This has now become part of the educational training pathway of that particular professional group. However, it was recognised that the model of leadership competence applied equally to all other clinical professions and the Clinical Leadership Competency Framework (CLCF) was produced from the MLCF to meet this need.

The CLCF is the focus of this text offering an emphasis on the multi-professional practice of NHS teams, recognising the contribution (clinical and in terms of leadership) that all professional groups can provide to the benefit of patient care.

A framework for this book

This book has been written as a text for trainees, tutors and practitioners. There are case studies throughout to support the text and assist the reader.

In Chapter 2 we outline the structure of the Clinical Leadership Competency Framework, the background to its development, the design and how to use it.

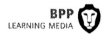

Chapter 3 then opens into a general discussion about the debate and evolution of approaches to leadership. Is it management? Or are these terms distinct and separate and what is the relationship between the two? What are the different approaches, styles and traits of leadership?

In Chapter 4 we describe the relationship between good leadership and organisational performance and suggest that all clinicians can make an enhanced contribution to improved patient care and to overall organisational performance by developing and utilising the skill set within the CLCF. This is elaborated further in Chapter 5 in the context of patient safety.

Given the past difficulties in achieving widespread embedding of leadership behaviours in the workforce, in Chapter 6, we describe the vital role that regulators, higher education institutions and the profession's representative bodies, such as colleges and societies, can play in promoting this aim and the work being undertaken to achieve it.

The ability to exercise leadership is very dependent on the context of the individual and this varies dependent on their career stage. Chapters 7–10 are designed to assist the learner understand leadership and its application in some contexts – ward, community/ primary care, clinic or other service setting. The case studies contributed here have come from practitioners working at various levels and roles. They represent their stories and how they have linked leadership and clinical service delivery.

Chapter 11 is specifically for tutors as they provide the crucial grounding for the acquisition of leadership skills throughout the clinicians care path.

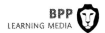

Chapter references

Edmonstone, J. Clinical Leadership: The Elephant in the Room. *International Journal of Health Planning and Management* 2009; 24: 290–305

Spurgeon, P C, and Klaber, R (2011) *Medical Leadership: A practical guide for tutors and trainees*. First Edition. London: BPP Learning Media.

Storey, John, and Holti, Richard, (2013). Possibilities and pitfalls for clinical leadership in improving service quality, innovation and productivity. Final report. NIHR Service Delivery and Organisation programme, HMSO, London, United Kingdom.

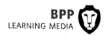

Chapter 2

The Clinical Leadership Competency Framework

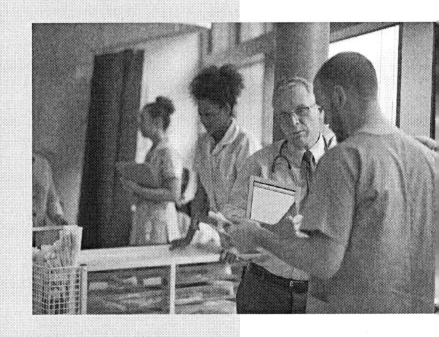

The Clinical Leadership Competency Framework

Chapter overview

This chapter provides:

- A background to the development of the Clinical Leadership Competency Framework (CLCF).

- A description of the CLCF and how it applies to clinicians and their training.

- The design of the CLCF and how it relates to different career stages.

Introduction

There are many examples of poor practice and system failure within health and social care where a lack of leadership – at an individual, collective and organisation level – has been identified as an important factor. For example, the two reports by Robert Francis into the Mid Staffordshire Foundation Trust make recommendations on professional leadership and the quality assurance of staff training (Department of Health, 2010; The Mid Staffordshire NHS Foundation Trust Public Inquiry, 2013). Failure to provide safe and appropriate care, treatment and support for residents at Winterbourne View care home has led the regulator, the Care Quality Commission (CQC), to launch a programme of unannounced inspections into similar services.

An effective response to these and other challenges facing health and social care provision can only be achieved if the critical role of leadership is recognised and addressed. Clinicians need to be not only experts in their chosen clinical discipline, but possess competent leadership and management skills that enable them to be more actively involved in the planning, delivery and transformation of services for patients.

Work to develop and build leadership capability and capacity within the workforce has been underway for many years within the National Health Service (NHS) and healthcare, and is now gaining momentum in adult social care services.

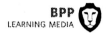

In healthcare, the Leadership Framework (LF) was published in July 2011. It has five core domains plus two additional domains designed for the most senior leaders and covers the four stages of leadership development from Own Practice/Immediate Team through to Whole Organisation/Healthcare System (Department of Health, 2011). It is a universal model such that all staff can contribute to the leadership task where and when their expertise and qualities are relevant and appropriate to the context in which they work. Not everyone is necessarily a leader but everyone can contribute to the leadership process by exercising leadership behaviours.

A key component of the Leadership Framework is the CLCF, which has been designed to be applicable throughout the United Kingdom and applies to every clinician at all stages of their career (Department of Health, 2011).

The CLCF itself is derived from the original Medical Leadership Competency Framework (MLCF) developed as a product of the Enhancing Engagement in Medical Leadership undertaken by the Institute of Innovation and Improvement and the Academy of Medical Royal Colleges (between 2005 to 2011) (NHS Institute for Innovation and Improvement and Academy of Medical Royal Colleges, 2010).

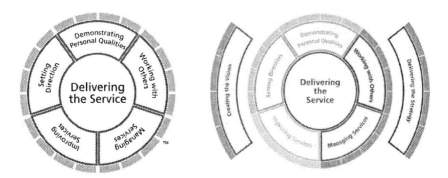

Clinical/Medical Leadership   Leadership Framework
Competency Framework

Figure 2.1 The five domains of the CLCF and the MLCF shown in Figure 2.1 form the basis of the expanded Leadership Framework.

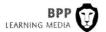

Background to the development of the CLCF

In January 2010 the Clinical Leadership work stream of the National Leadership Council (NLC) commissioned the NHS Institute for Innovation and Improvement (NHS Institute) to test the applicability of the generic leadership competences in the Medical Leadership Competency Framework (MLCF) for the other regulated clinical professions (National Leadership Council, 2010).

The aim of this was to work with the clinical professions to build leadership awareness and capability across the health service, by embedding leadership competencies in undergraduate education, postgraduate training and continuing professional development.

Ninety-seven people from fifty-one organisations representing the clinical professions, their regulatory bodies, policy makers and the higher education sector were interviewed.

The findings of the CLCF project demonstrated a recognition that leadership is important, and the need to further develop leadership capability within the clinical professions, is unquestioned (Long *et al*; 2011).

The level of interest was high amongst all the clinical professions and there was an overall willingness to adopt the CLCF. Practitioners embraced the concept of the Leadership Framework because it afforded a common and consistent approach to development based on their shared professional values and beliefs, which is nested within the domains and standards of their professional bodies rather than organisational structures which are ever changing.

Coverage of leadership within existing training and curricula within the professions

Long *et al's* research also demonstrated that leadership and management competences within existing education and training were varyingly described, applied and assessed, and tended to focus on the practitioner rather than the wider systems in which they function; they were rarely described as leadership standards or competences. There was no single national leadership curriculum or framework for non-medical clinicians and higher education institutions tend to relate their content to the minimum or threshold standards set down by the relevant regulator as well the professional body's guidance.

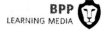

There was also very little, if any, consistent assessment of leadership capability in the professions or in regulation, education or workforce. Where assessment processes existed, there was no standard or framework that prescribed how it should be uniformly developed or undertaken.

The project team also found that the private sector players, the larger private sector firms with high street outlets, and bodies representing the private sector, were interested in developing leadership capacity within their workforce.

The findings revealed widespread support for a common approach to leadership development across the professional, regulatory and education sectors and the NHS. The willingness of the professions and the practitioners is very important, however, there are broader system-wide considerations – regulatory, education and workforce – that are equally important and without which the professional bodies would find it difficult to adopt and embed the CLCF (Long & Spurgeon, 2012).

The Clinical Leadership Competency Framework

Clinicians train and work in many settings and sectors. The CLCF is applicable across the United Kingdom and has been developed through consultation with a wide cross section of staff, patients, professional bodies and academics. Its development also had the input of all the clinical professional bodies and has the support of the chief professions officers, the professions advisory boards, the peak education bodies and the Department of Health.

The CLCF is designed to be read and used in conjunction with the relevant professional and service documents provided by the professional bodies, government bodies, regulators and higher education institutions as described in Chapter 6.

Leadership and clinicians

People understand the term 'leadership' in many different ways. Perhaps the most common stereotypic idea is of the individual, powerful, charismatic leader with followers clearly in subordinate roles. Such situations do exist but are quite limited, rather outdated

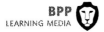

and by the very rarity of charismatic qualities make it a poor model for leadership development. This way of thinking tends to focus on the individual as a leader rather than the processes of leadership.

A more modern conceptualisation sees leadership as something to be used by all but at different levels where exemplar clinical leadership is less about pushing the way forward and more about creating a cohesive team working to a common goal (Grint & Holt, 2011). Effective responsible leaders need also be equally effective responsible clinical followers (Long & Spurgeon, 2012).

This model of leadership is often described as shared, or distributed, leadership and is especially appropriate where tasks are more complex and highly interdependent – as in healthcare (Conger & Pearce, 2003) see figure 2.2. Not everyone is necessarily a leader but everyone can contribute to the leadership process by using the behaviours described in the five core domains of the CLCF: demonstrating personal qualities, working with others, managing services, improving services, and setting direction (figure 2.3).

As a model it emphasises the responsibility of all practising clinicians to seek to contribute to the leadership process and to develop and empower the leadership capacity of colleagues.

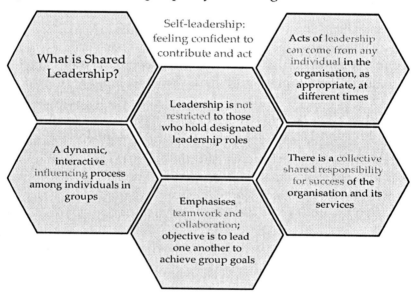

Figure 2.2 The concept of shared leadership

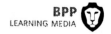

Design

Delivering services to patients, service users, carers and the public is at the heart of the Clinical Leadership Competency Framework. Clinicians work hard to improve services for people.

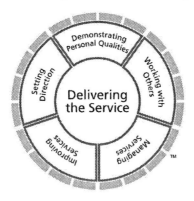

Figure 2.3 The Clinical Leadership Competency Framework

The word 'patient' is used generically to cover patients, service users, and all those who receive healthcare. The word 'other' is used to describe all colleagues from any discipline and organisation, as well as patients, service users, carers and the public.

The five domains of the CLCF are highlighted below. To improve the quality and safety of health and care services, it is essential that clinicians are competent in each of the five leadership domains.

Domain 1. Demonstrating personal qualities – effective leadership requires individuals to draw upon their values, strengths and abilities to deliver high standards of service.

This requires them to demonstrate effectiveness in the following elements:

1.1   Developing self-awareness
1.2   Managing yourself
1.3   Continuing personal development
1.4   Acting with integrity

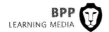

Domain 2. Working with others – effective leadership requires individuals to work with others in teams and networks to deliver and improve services.

This requires them to demonstrate effectiveness in the following elements:

2.1 Developing networks
2.2 Building and maintaining relationships
2.3 Encouraging contribution
2.4 Working within teams

Domain 3. Managing services – effective leadership requires individuals to focus on the success of the organisation(s) in which they work.

This requires them to demonstrate effectiveness in the following elements:

3.1 Planning
3.2 Managing resources
3.3 Managing people
3.4 Managing performance

Domain 4. Improving services – effective leadership requires individuals to make a real difference to people's health by delivering high quality services and by developing improvements to services.

This requires them to demonstrate effectiveness in the following elements:

4.1 Ensuring patient safety
4.2 Critically evaluating
4.3 Encouraging improvement and innovation
4.4 Facilitating transformation

Domain 5. Setting direction – effective leadership requires individuals to contribute to the strategy and aspirations of the organisation and act in a manner consistent with its values.

This requires them to demonstrate effectiveness in the following elements:

5.1 Identifying the contexts for change
5.2 Applying knowledge and evidence
5.3 Making decisions
5.4 Evaluating impact

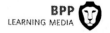

Within each domain there are four categories called elements and each of these elements is further divided into four competency statements which describe the activity or outcomes all clinicians should be able to demonstrate.

For example:

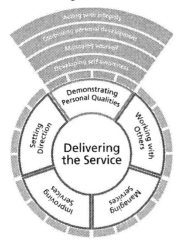

Domain 1: Demonstrating personal qualities

Effective leaders need to draw upon their values, strengths and abilities to deliver high standards of care.

This requires leaders to demonstrate competence in the areas of:

Figure 2.4 Demonstrating Personal Qualities with 4 elements

Element 1.1 Developing self awareness

The competency statements for Element 1.1 are:

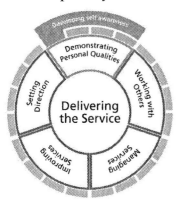

Figure 2.5 CLCF Demonstrating Personal Qualities, 1.1 Developing Self-Awareness

- Recognise and articulate their own values and principles, understanding how these may differ from those of other individuals and groups.

- Identify their own strengths and limitations, the impact of their behaviour on others, and the effect of stress on their own behaviour.

- Identify their own emotions and prejudices and understand how these can affect their judgment and behaviour.

- Obtain, analyse and act on feedback from a variety of sources.

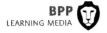

To assist the user to understand how they relate to the framework there are practical contextual examples in practice available for each element, plus examples of learning and development activity.

Who is the CLCF for?

The Clinical Leadership Competency Framework applies to every clinician at all stages of their professional journey – from the time they enter formal training, become qualified as a practitioner and throughout their continuing professional development as experienced practitioners.

There is no universal or common pathway followed by all of the clinical professions and the way a clinician demonstrates competence and ability will vary according to their career trajectory and their level of experience and training (Table 2.1). However, all competences should be capable of being achieved at all career stages, though at varying degrees dependant on the contexts.

Within the various developmental routes for each profession some core processes have been identified and are used throughout the CLCF. These are as:

- Student – pre-registration entry level formal education.
- Practitioner – qualified or registered professional.
- Experienced practitioner – practitioner with greater complexity and responsibility in their role.

Using this spectrum as a guide, examples are used throughout the CLCF to provide users with context in which they are able to relate their practice. All domains and elements of the CLCF are dynamic and apply to all students, clinicians in training, experienced practitioners and consultant practitioners. However, the application of and opportunity to demonstrate the competences in the CLCF will differ according to the career stage of the clinician and the type of role they fulfil. The context in which competence can be achieved will become more complex and demanding with career progression.

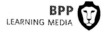

Student	For example all students will have access to relevant learning opportunities within a variety of situations including:
	• Peer interaction • Group learning • Clinical placements • Activities and responsibilities within the university • Involvement with charities, social groups and organisations
	All these situations can provide a clinical student with the opportunity to develop experience of leadership, their personal styles and abilities, and to understand how effective leadership will have a positive impact as they move from student to practitioner on graduating.
Practitioner	Qualified clinicians are very often the key person relating to patients and other staff, and are the ones who are experiencing how day-to-day healthcare works in action. They are also often undertaking more education and training to further consolidate and develop their skills and knowledge in everyday practice.
	Practitioners are uniquely placed to develop experience in management and leadership through relationships with other people, departments and ways of working and to understand how the patient experiences healthcare, and how the processes and systems of delivering care can be improved. Specific activities such as clinical audit and research also offer the opportunity to learn leadership and management skills. With all this comes the need to understand how their speciality and focus of care contributes to the wider healthcare system.

Experienced practitioner	Experienced practitioners hold more complex roles with greater responsibility. Clinicians need an understanding of the need for each area of the wider healthcare system to play its part. Experienced clinicians develop their abilities in leadership within their services and practices and by working with colleagues in other settings and on projects. Their familiarity with their specific focus of care enables them to work outside their immediate setting and to look further at ways to improve the experience of healthcare for patients and colleagues. As established members of staff or as partners, they are able to develop further their leadership abilities by actively contributing to the running of the organisation and to the way care is provided generally.

Table 2.1

How the CLCF can be applied and used

The CLCF will be used by the health and care organisations, professional bodies, educators and individuals to:

- Help with personal development planning and career progression.

- Help with the design and commissioning of formal training curricula and development programmes by colleges and societies, higher education institutions and public healthcare providers.

- Highlight individual strengths and development areas through self-assessment, appraisal and structured feedback from colleagues.

Students

For clinicians undertaking formal education and training their courses will cover a broad range of topics. It is important that leadership learning is incorporated within the mainstream curriculum, rather than regarded as something additional or even peripheral to that core.

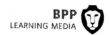

The underpinning practical and learning & development examples used throughout the CLCF provide students with context in which they are able to relate their practice and the type of development activity they can undertake to achieve each element.

Practitioners and experienced practitioners

When clinicians enter the workforce the CLCF can be used or adapted to help with professional development, such as continuing professional development (CPD), required or provided by their employer, society or college. It can also be used for staff appraisals, self-assessment and performance management.

Many of the learning and development opportunities identified at student level apply equally at practitioner or experienced practitioner level. The learning opportunities are consistent with good care provision, emphasising the CLCF as an integrated, rather than separate, set of behaviours.

The CLCF is designed to apply throughout a clinician's career. The NHS Leadership Framework, can also be used by clinicians to recognise their stage of leadership development in the context of other non-clinical colleagues. The Leadership Framework is the same as the CLCF in terms of the first five domains and offers generic workplace examples as well as two additional domains designed to support those in senior leadership roles, which may be helpful for clinicians aspiring to or already in these roles.

Most recent development in models of leadership

Healthcare Leadership Model

One aspect of the 2010 NHS reforms was the establishment of a new Leadership Academy. Although the NHS Leadership Framework was only published in 2011, the Academy decided that a revision was needed. The swell of concern about the failings at Mid-Staffordshire NHS Foundation Trust may have prompted a need to be seen to be responding. The logic of the arguments which were put forward for a revision is genuinely hard to follow. The first was that the current Leadership Framework had failed to prevent the problems

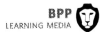

at Mid-Staffordshire, and yet the Framework charged with this failure had not been in existence at the time and indeed had not been implemented until well after the Mid-Staffordshire problems.

Secondly, it was suggested that the dominant command-and-control culture, with matching management mechanisms and styles, was confusing, with the Framework's emphasis upon collaboration and shared leadership.

Cases of over-dominant chief executives on Trust Boards (Storey et al; 2010), and NHS managers being too reliant on 'pace-setting' – that is, an over-reliance on demanding targets, leading from the front, and a reluctance to delegate (Santry, 2011) – has led to a shift in emphasis towards autonomy, responsibility and accountability in the UK and countries such as Australia.

The King's Fund has called for a move away from the pace-setting, command-and-control, and target-driven approach, and there is, arguably, a need to bring more to the foreground the social purpose and meaningful contribution of NHS and NHS-funded organisations.

Again, it is not entirely clear whether the new model is advocating shared leadership as the key future focus or trying to explain the apparent perceived contradiction between shared leadership and personal accountability.

The thinking underpinning the development of the NHS Leadership Model has been stated as intending to deal with the duality of shared leadership forms, while also clarifying the behaviours expected of those occupying leadership positions in the NHS. More practically, as shown in Figure 2.6, the desire to promote greater congruence between the leadership behaviours, the needs of the customer and improving organisational performance.

Perhaps the key backdrop and trigger for a review of existing leadership models was the launch by the Leadership Academy of a suite of traditional individual-participant programmes sponsored and organised by the Academy.

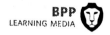

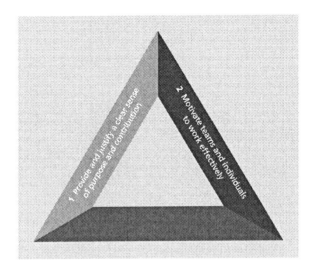

Figure 2.6 Focus on Improving system performance

Source: Storey, J and Holti, R, Towards a New Model of Leadership for the NHS, NHS Leadership Academy, June 2013.

The Design of the NHS Healthcare Leadership Model

The Healthcare Leadership Model (NHS Model) is made up of nine 'leadership dimensions'. Like the CLCF, personal qualities are an important part of the NHS Model; being aware of your strengths and limitations in these areas will have a direct effect on how you behave and interact with others, and they with you. Clinicians working positively on their personal qualities will lead to a focus on care and high-quality services for patients and service users, their carers, and their families. Within the NHS Model, personal qualities are dispersed throughout the relevant dimensions rather than an explicit domain such as in the CLCF.

For each dimension within the NHS Model, leadership behaviours are shown on a four-part scale which ranges from essential through proficient, and strong to exemplary. Although the complexity and sophistication of the behaviours increase as the user moves up the scale, the scale is not tied to particular job roles or levels. So people in junior roles may find themselves to be within the strong or exemplary parts of the scale, and senior staff may find themselves in the essential or proficient parts. Similarly, you may find where you judge yourself to be may vary depending on the

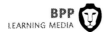

dimension itself. For example, you may be mostly 'strong' in a few dimensions, exemplary in one, and essential or proficient in others. This may be appropriate depending on your job role, or it may show that there are areas that need some development or that are a particular strength.

Within these scales, the leadership behaviours themselves are presented as a series of questions. The questions are short descriptions of what the leadership dimension looks like at each part of the scale.

The NHS Leadership Model and the CLCF are very closely related. Like the MLCF, the CLCF has been designed specifically for clinicians. The CLCF is a practical descriptor of the NHS Model. Many individuals, organisations and programmes have worked hard to integrate the CLCF domains, elements, and behavioural indicators into their work and there is no change planned for the CLCF.

Chapter summary

In this chapter we learned:

- The importance of frontline clinicians having the leadership capability to meet the challenges in today's healthcare.

- The ability to manage and influence change is vital.

- Promoting leadership development is necessary for all clinical professions that work in healthcare.

- Leadership competences will be incorporated into education and training.

Three things to try

1. Read the CLCF and reflect on how your practice changes dependent on the context you are working in.

2. Start applying the learning and development examples.

3. Identify your leadership development needs using the CLCF self-assessment tool http://www.leadershipacademy.nhs.uk/wp-content/uploads/2012/11/NHSLeadership-Framework-CLCFSelfAssessmentTool.pdf

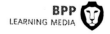

Chapter references

Conger, A J and Pearce, C L. (2003). *Shared Leadership: reframing the how's and why's of leadership.* Sage.

Department of Health. (2010). *The Mid Staffordshire NHS Foundation Trust Inquiry*, Department of Health Gate Reference 13743.

Department of Health (2011) *The Clinical Leadership Competency Framework.* Coventry. NHS Institute for Innovation and Improvement.

Department of Health (2011) *The Leadership Framework.* Coventry. NHS Institute for Innovation and Improvement.

Grint K, Holt, C. *Followership in the NHS: A report for The King's Fund Commission on Leadership and Management in the NHS 2011.* [Online] Available at HYPERLINK "http://www.kingsfund.org.uk/leadershipcommission"www.kingsfund.org.uk/leadershipcommission [Accessed 23.07.12].

Long, P, W et al. The CLCF: developing leadership capacity and capability in the clinical professions. *International Journal of Clinical Leadership 2009;* 17 (2).

Long P, W and Spurgeon, P, C. Embedding leadership into professional, regulatory and educational standards. *International Journal of Clinical Leadership* 2012; 17, (4).

National Leadership Council (2010). *Report on the findings of the Clinical Leadership Competency Framework Project.* Coventry. NHS Institute for Innovation and Improvement.

NHS Institute for Innovation and Improvement and Academy of Medical Royal Colleges (2010) *Medical Leadership Competency Framework*, 3rd edition, Coventry: NHS Institute for Innovation and Improvement.

The Mid Staffordshire NHS Foundation Trust Public Inquiry (2013) *Report of the Mid Staffordshire NHS Foundation Trust Public Inquiry*, House of Commons. 6 Feb 2013. The Stationery Office, London.

NHS Leadership Academy (2013) *The Healthcare Leadership Model*, version 1.0, Leeds England: NHS Leadership Academy.

Santry, C. (2011). *'Resilient NHS managers lack required leadership skills DH research says.'* Health Service Journal. 6 July.

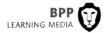

Storey J, Holti R, Bate P Salaman G, Winchester N, and Green R. (2010). *The Intended and Unintended Outcomes of New Governance Arrangements within the NHS. Final Report for the National Co-ordinating Centre for NHS Service Delivery and Organisation R&D (NCCSDO) SDO Research project 08/1618/129.*

Storey J, Holti, R (2013) *Towards a New Model of Leadership for the NHS. NHS Leadership Academy, Leeds, England. Jun. 2013 [Online] Available at* www.leadershipacademy.nhs.uk/wp-content/uploads/2013/05/Towards-a-New-Model-of-Leadership-2013.pdf

The authors acknowledge the kind permission by the NHS Leadership Academy to use the graphics for the Clinical Leadership Competency Framework and Leadership Framework in Chapter 2.

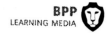

Chapter 3
Management and leadership

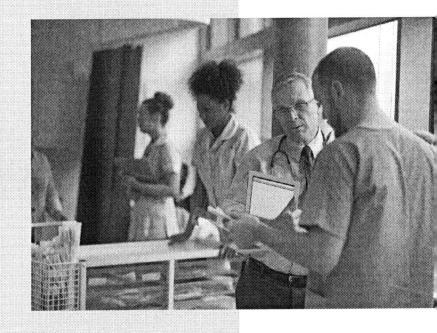

Management and leadership

Chapter overview

This chapter provides:

- A discussion of the distinction between management and leadership.

- An understanding of the various models and approaches to leadership.

- An explanation of the model of shared leadership that underpins the Clinical Leadership Competency Framework.

Introduction

The previous chapter introduced the reader to the importance of clinical leadership together with the evolution and content of the CLCF. For many years the term clinical management has been quite prevalent with individuals described as going on a management course or moving from clinical work to become a manager. However, the CLCF like its forerunner the Medical Leadership Competency Framework (MLCF) uses the term leadership.

How far does this represent the replacement of one term by another, or is it simply usage of a more fashionable word? It is possible too that it could be a source of confusion and misunderstanding. Certainly it is not unusual in a presentation on this topic for a member of the audience to ask 'Ah but are you really talking about management or leadership?'

There are two issues here:

- Should management be clearly differentiated from leadership?

- When we use the term leadership are we (authors, commentators and readers) all using it to mean exactly the same thing?

A number of well-established texts discuss these issues at length; see Hartley & Benington (2010) *'Leadership for Healthcare'* or Spurgeon, Clark & Ham (2011) *'Medical Leadership: from the dark side to centre stage'*. It is not the intention here to go into great depth. The overall aim of this book is to support practice in the use and implementation of the CLCF. However, as questions about the two concepts may arise it is perhaps worth being armed with a few discussion points.

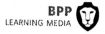
BPP
LEARNING MEDIA

Management or leadership

Apart from the question of is it possible to draw a clear distinction between the two terms there is of course the larger question of does it matter? It seems that it may do in terms of what assumptions people make about the two concepts and how this might affect their willingness to participate in them. Traditionally the NHS was seen as an administered service, supporting the delivery of care by clinical staff. The managerialism of the 1980s and 1990s proved somewhat divisive as it sought to establish managerial accountability, as some would describe it, over clinical staff. More recently the model has been to seek to invite all staff groups to contribute within a broad concept of leadership. On the whole this has proved rather more attractive with an increasingly strong emphasis on clinical leadership. It would seem then that a distinction between management and leadership can matter, at least in terms of how people perceive it.

A stereotype of managers, or management, probably plays into this perspective with individuals feeling slightly resentful about being managed and seeing management as inherently bureaucratic and controlling. In contrast the notion of a charismatic leader articulating an inspiring vision of the future is rather more appealing.

The literature is distinctly unhelpful with some authors listing various functions of management or leadership and thereby implying that they are different. Other authors simply don't attempt to resolve the issue at all. Yuki (2006) captures the conundrum quite nicely when suggesting that most studies of leadership 'are conducted on people who call themselves managers, so presumably they are leaders as well'.

Spurgeon & Cragg (2007) suggest that the focus may in part be determined by the context in which an organisation functions. They say 'the basic functions of management- planning, budgeting, organising, controlling resources and problem solving- are vital for the smooth running of any organisation: without them anarchy may result. These managerial activities though are most appropriate when organisations and the society around them are stable and relatively predictable. The constant and continual change occurring in society and the NHS goes some way to explaining why such a premium is placed on leadership. If organisations need to adapt and change to new circumstances then leaders who challenge, motivate and inspire others towards a new vision are critical.

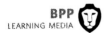

Perhaps a simplistic summary perspective might be that managers are primarily concerned with making the current systems and its procedures operate as efficiently and effectively as possible. Leaders on the whole seek to change what currently exists so that the organisation will be better equipped to deal with the future.

The interrelations of leadership and management

The position adopted here and implicit in the CLCF is that there is a merging of the two functions, largely driven by the context or situation and that a hard and fast distinction is unhelpful. It can lead to the assignment of labels where someone is described as a manager or a leader, clearly segregating the roles and often maintaining a rather fixed position. The following examples may help to make the argument that any distinction between the two terms quickly becomes blurred in practice.

Organisations will often undertake significant reorganisation of their practices and procedures with operating changes implied for many staff. The responsibility for the implementation programme will typically fall to a manager and yet the success of the project will often turn on the manager's ability to communicate and convince other staff of the merits of accepting new tasks and ways of working. The key ingredient is that of influencing others and this is said to be a critical component of leadership. It may be that some managers find this influencing role very challenging and are not particularly good at it. Such a performance deficit may, for that manager, mark a dividing line between their capacity as a manager and their potential to develop and perform as a leader. The blurring of the task in this example is clear with aspects of management (planning, scheduling, monitoring) but equally leadership aspects (communicating, influencing, motivating).

In another example it may be that a relatively junior clinician may want to improve or change the way a service is provided. This may well involve various aspects of communication, talking to and influencing colleagues and managers. These processes are reasonably viewed as aspects of leadership. However, it is almost certain that in very short order the clinician will be asked to prepare a business plan to demonstrate the viability of the

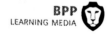

proposed service improvement. Few would dispute that the business planning process is a classic management task and so again we see leadership and management activities soon overlapping. The point is that most significant tasks in organisations require aspects of management and leadership. Individuals may at different times focus upon one aspect more than another and some may find the transition difficult. But it is not just managers who may struggle to encompass leadership.

Equally some leaders may be able to articulate an inspirational vision but are not good at putting in place an operational plan to achieve the goal. As Spurgeon & Cragg (2007) conclude it may be better to think of management and leadership as processes which interact and support each other and are both necessary for effective organisations; however at specific times one may be emphasised more than the other.

Approaches to leadership

Is it just academic pedantry to question whether the term leadership is always used clearly and unambiguously? Or is it actually important in practice to have greater precision and clarity about the term? At a fairly simple level, the definition of leadership may well have implications. Quite frequently trainers and educators will comment that 'everyone can be a leader', or 'leadership is the responsibility of everyone'. Some people hearing this type of statement will, by choice or some sense of self-insight, immediately think 'I am not a leader; I don't want to be.' This quite simple example contains a number of concepts of leadership, which may result in some individuals construing leadership as not for them. It is likely that such individuals will have a rather traditional and stereotypical view of leadership as involving a charismatic, inspirational commanding figure who carries others along by his/her sheer presence. They will then conclude – and probably quite rightly – that they are therefore not a leader. However, this is potentially an inappropriate conclusion, because it is grounded in their particular model of leadership. Therefore it is worth a brief detour into the nature of leadership and the approaches to describing it. Hopefully this will equip the reader with the knowledge and information to understand and perhaps challenge certain statements about leadership.

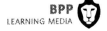

Leadership models

The study of leadership has existed for many years and has been consistently documented and added to since the 1920s. A particular concern has been with leadership effectiveness, with practitioners seeking answers about the ingredients of success to academics attempting to understand how to demonstrate the impact of leadership. The search to understand leadership has followed a path shaped to a large extent by the nature of society around it at the time. Initially, the focus was on the individual and sought to describe the traits of great successful leaders, reflecting the individualism of entrepreneurship. It then moved to more behavioural approaches, documenting what leaders did, which itself was extended to incorporate details of the context or situation in which leadership occurred. More recently, as society became more complex, democratic and collective, so leadership models attempted to incorporate aspects of complexity and to reflect the impact of education on breaking down conventional social hierarchies. (Please see Northouse (2010), and Hartley & Benington (2010) for good reviews of leadership models). Many definitions can be found in such texts but the following simple, workable one will be used here: when you boil it all down, contemporary leadership seems to be a matter of aligning people towards common goals and empowering them to take the actions needed to reach them.

Trait theory

The earliest conceptualisation of leadership focused on trying to identify the traits/characteristics of individuals who, by status, power, achievement, or some form of recognition, were deemed to be leaders. This approach assumed such individuals possessed the vital ingredients that made them leaders. If this could be identified and described it would enable the right people (ie leaders) to be appointed to the appropriate leadership roles. An implicit assumption was that the necessary characteristics would see the same people emerge as leaders across a range of different situations – because they possessed the essential qualities whilst others did not. This theory also regarded these characteristics as innate; people simply had them or did not. Despite decades of research in pursuit of the key characteristics, the approach has been relatively unsuccessful. Only a few factors (eg superior intelligence, self-confidence, self-starter, extrovert)

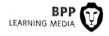

emerged with any stability across different research contexts. As products of a considerable amount of research, these findings are actually quite meagre and could probably have been specified at the outset. The trait theory, though, lingers partly because people still use their stereotypical model of leadership to judge whether others could be potential leaders, and also because there seems to be some sort of comfort factor in believing in the great leader who will come along and put everything right. This perspective can be seen in the searches conducted by large organisations for a new Chief Executive to restore the fortunes of an ailing company. Recently, Alimo-Metcalfe (2001) developed a more modern and sophisticated model of the trait approach, in her description of engaging leadership. The focus of such work has shifted from the great leader to a more collaborative, participative style, but remains nonetheless a set of character descriptions. The trait theory has produced many lists of qualities, which tend to overlap and universally fail to deal with a number of key questions:

- Are all the characteristics needed in all contexts?

- What combinations are required in particular circumstances?

- How much of any quality does an individual need to possess, can great strength in one area compensate for another?

- How in the context of a selection process will classic qualities such as integrity (worthy as it may be) be assessed?

The final deficiencies of the approach stem from the implicit assumption that such characteristics are innate and therefore are largely unable to be acquired. Therefore, if someone does not seem to possess all or certain traits, can they aspire to a leadership role or not? It is also particularly difficult to know what to do with such lists of characteristics.

Because of the lack of specificity, how can an individual reconcile positive feelings about some qualities, with negative ones about others? Is it possible to develop the missing characteristics if they are largely regarded as innate? Perhaps the most optimistic and reasonable conclusion is that as it is clear leaders do emerge, then the range of qualities described are probably relevant to some extent; and that leaders will possess a wide variety of combinations of these personal qualities. On this basis, it is possible that everyone can contribute as a leader, but in different ways, with different approaches and by using varying qualities. However, this is unsatisfactory as a research conclusion to an area of study.

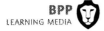

Leadership style and context

The relative failure of the personality- or trait-based model saw a shift in focus from who leaders are to what they do, and the importance of the context in which leadership occurs. Key categories of behaviour which emerged from this strand of research focused on the following:

- Task behaviours: giving a priority to getting the job done.
- Relationship behaviours: emphasising the way people work together.

The combination and emphasis given to each of these resulted in the concept of leadership styles, with debates about whether task and relationship styles could be found in one person alone, or, if necessary, could be fulfilled by separate people. For example, extremely task-focused individuals (often much valued for their level of achievement) will often ride roughshod over the feelings and concerns of others in order to ensure goals are achieved. A more supportive, concerned style was considered to be incompatible with task-achievement and almost impossible to provide simultaneously. However, there is little clear support for these perspectives and indeed a very modern conceptualisation of leadership would now suggest that a supportive, participative style can be the basis of promoting organisational achievement. The aspiration of this research was to link a particular style to outcome, so that the most effective style could be identified; suitable individuals could be offered training and development so that they could work in this way. Once more, however, no such clear relationship could be established. Instead, the inconsistency of results relating to leadership styles led to a belief that it was the variation in context that held the key. This has been described as the situational or contingency model of leadership. There is a slight difference of emphasis but crucially the idea was that the behaviour of the leader would be more or less appropriate and effective, depending on certain aspects of the context. The degree of competence of the members of the team being led, the rewards available to this follower group and the complexity of the task itself are particularly relevant factors. There has been value in understanding the impact of a range of factors on the success of leadership behaviours but it is also fair to say that in trying to establish a degree of certainty about specific leadership related factors the dynamic inter-play of too many influences has proved rather too complex for clear results.

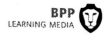

Transactional vs. Transformational

Quite a strong strand of leadership work has formed around the concept of transactional versus transformational leadership. Aspects of both concepts were presented in earlier parts of this chapter, both in the discussion of management and leadership and of task or relationship-based leadership styles. Transactional leadership is seen as part of a series of exchanges or transactions between a leader and followers, normally based in a hierarchical organisational structure.

In contrast, transformational leadership does not depend on hierarchy but is a product of followers' desire and willingness to be led by a particular individual. Transformational leadership is based on a personal connection affording influence. As later versions of the transactional/transformational model began to describe, the two are not unlike the managerial (transactional)/leadership (transformational) dimension described earlier; Bass (1999) has described them as being on a continuum. Transformational leadership is generally regarded as the style essential to changing and improving organisations; it has also been associated with greater staff satisfaction, motivation and performance. However, the model still represents an underlying conceptualisation of leadership as based around the individual. A recent model has sought to take a more collective approach to leadership. It is referred to as shared or distributed leadership and is probably the most persuasive of modern strands.

Shared, collective or distributed leadership

The leadership literature is increasingly recognising that the leader-centric model, where all the focus is on one person, is quite limited. The increasingly complex set of tasks facing organisations has seen a growing reliance on teams; here, leadership tasks are shared across teams, organisational boundaries and networks. Each team member's individual experience, knowledge and capacity is valued and used to distribute or share the job of leadership through the team, in response to each context or challenge being faced. Implicit in this is a realisation that it is unrealistic for one individual to have all the necessary skills. The approach is also inherently more democratic ie it recognises that in a society with higher levels of education, more individuals will be capable of a leadership contribution.

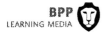

The burgeoning interest in shared leadership chimes well with flatter, less hierarchical organisations which need to respond rapidly and flexibly to continuing change. It gives rise to the advocated position that everyone can make a contribution as a leader at their appropriate level in the organisation. Furthermore, it makes the vital point that is crucial to this entire text: it makes more sense to talk of leadership rather than of a leader. Leadership consists of a range of behaviours described in the CLCF. These behaviours can be acquired and used at any level in the organisation, and therefore all can contribute leadership (as opposed to leaders) within the relevant part of their organisation.

The CLCF is built upon this model of shared leadership. It is aimed at ensuring that all clinical professions can contribute leadership behaviours as the task and content demands, and as their level in the organisation allows.

Chapter summary

In this chapter we learned:

- The distinction between management and leadership and how the two concepts work together.

- A stereotype of managers, or management, being seen as inherently bureaucratic and controlling.

- Personality or character driven models of leadership have been replaced by more collective approaches.

- It makes more sense to think of leadership than leader, which is shared with all being able to contribute leadership behaviours as the task and context demands, and as their level within the organisation allows.

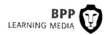

Three things to try

1. Think about a time when it is necessary to exercise both leadership and management action.

2. Review a recurring issue you have and how working with others can be applied to achieve a different outcome.

3. Try facilitating a multi-disciplinary approach to an issue where colleagues take on the role of other disciplines, or patients or carers.

Chapter references

Alimo-Metcalfe, B and Alban-Metcalfe, T. The development of a new transformational leadership questionnaire. *Journal of Occupational and Organisational Psychology.* 2001; 74, 1–27.

Bass. B. (1999). *Two decades of research & development in transformational leadership.* European Journal of Work & Organisational Psychology 12, 47–59.

Hartley J and Benington J (2010). *Leadership for Healthcare.* Bristol, UK: The Policy Press.

Northouse P, G (2010). *Leadership: Theory and Practice.* 5th edition. Thousand Oaks, CA: Sage.

Spurgeon, P and Cragg, R (2007). *Is it management or leadership?* In Chambers R, Mohanna K, Spurgeon P and Wall D (eds) 'How to Succeed as a Leader'. Oxford: Radcliffe Press.

Spurgeon P, Clark J and Ham C (2011) *Medical Leadership: From the Dark Side to Centre Stage.* Oxford: Radcliffe Press.

Yuki. G. (2006). *Leadership in organisations.* 6th Edition. Upper Sadle, NJ. Prentice Hall.

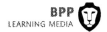

Chapter 3

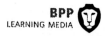

Chapter 4

The CLCF, patient care & organisational performance

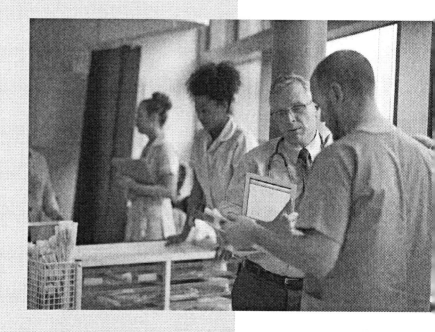

The CLCF, patient care & organisational performance

Chapter overview

This chapter provides:

- The relationship between leadership and good quality patient care.

- An analysis of how leadership may have an impact within healthcare organisations.

- An understanding of how individuals (clinicians) can make a contribution to the leadership process irrespective of their level of seniority and personal characteristics.

Introduction

Previous chapters have introduced the reader to the Clinical Leadership Competency Framework, described its origins and located the shared leadership model amongst the various models and approaches to management and leadership. In Chapter 5 we describe the crucial role that educational institutions and professional bodies can play in promoting and supporting clinicians to acquire the various competencies identified. The position of the authors is quite explicit in that all clinicians can make an enhanced contribution to improved patient care and to overall organisational performance by developing and utilising the skill set within the CLCF. Is this proposition just a belief, part of the rhetoric around clinical leadership or is there a basis of evidence on which the argument is made? This chapter considers some examples and evidence of where clinical leadership can make a difference.

Clinical leadership: potential impact

The case could probably begin and end with reference to the recent enquiry into the care deficiencies at Mid-Staffordshire NHS Foundation Trust (Francis Report, 2013). The lengthy report contains sad and disturbing accounts of poor care, but it is equally heavily populated with attributions to a failure of clinical leadership. The

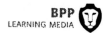

nursing profession has largely borne the brunt of this criticism and there has been much commentary and speculation about how the situation has arisen.

There is probably no single cause but as one is made aware of what did not happen or where accountability was not shown it is evident that if the behaviours represented in the CLCF had been demonstrated by more staff then certainly some of the problems may have been avoided. Patient care therefore is an immediate causality of a lack of good leadership skills in various clinical staff.

At a more conceptual, research based level Hartley & Benington (2010) offer what they describe as a value stream analysis of how leadership may have an impact within healthcare organisations. The possibilities are listed under a series of headings (some examples are given from Hartley & Benington, (2010)).

Inputs – leadership influence upon aspects such as recruitment and selection, financial resources available.

Activities – leadership may influence systems and procedures, teamwork, attitudes and culture.

Outputs – productivity, quality systems.

User Satisfaction – leadership may influence both patient and public perception of the work done in the organisation.

A number of research papers will provide supportive evidence under these broad headings. For example Vandenberghe *et al* (2002) found transformational leadership to be associated with higher levels of job satisfaction and reduced intention to leave. Ovretveit (2005) concludes that senior leadership is critical for service improvement. Shipton *et al* (2008) working with a large sample of staff (over 17,000) found good leaders to be associated with a range of performance ratings.

The value of clinical leadership is further reinforced when linked to a similar but slightly different concept of engagement. Spurgeon *et al* (2011) developed this concept in relation to medical engagement. They demonstrated that NHS Trusts with a high degree of medical engagement have higher levels of performance across a range of areas (patient experience, utilisation of resources, quality measures and patient safety). Macleod & Clarke (2009) looked at the notion of engagement across a range of sectors and staff groups. They

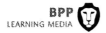

cite once again several studies that suggest enhanced engagement in organisation-wide goals is of benefit to the individual (Black, 2008), as well as the organisation itself. They see the role of leaders in promoting greater clinical engagement as vital.

The nature of clinical leadership

The evidence presented accords with a growing sense of the importance of clinical leadership. There is though relatively little discussion about what is meant by clinical leadership and whether it has distinctive characteristics. In respect of nursing leadership Lett (2002) argues that there has been an over-focus on senior leaders holding designated leadership roles, to the exclusion of those in more practice based positions. Whilst Stanley (2009) suggests that the constant turmoil in the NHS has led similarly to an over fixation on transformational leadership in nursing with little attention paid to alternative models. He goes on in a large study of perceptions of clinical leaders to advocate a model which he calls congruent leadership. Essentially this seems to describe leaders who by their actions and clinical care demonstrate and embody the values they wish to see in all clinical staff. Once again we see following the Francis Report (2013) an upsurge in interest in recruiting and developing individuals coming into health care professions around the values they hold.

Irrespective of the particular model followed it is time to say that whilst there have been very effective leaders drawn from the nursing and allied health professionals they have been in relatively short supply (Butterworth, 2009). This is perhaps especially true of non-nursing professions. It seems to have been the case that most of these groups have not seen leadership as a relevant development path. Given the high level of entry requirement now needed to train in many of these professional groups it is a serious waste of potential. As with doctors it may be that a rather false perspective of management of being about money and control that has inhibited interest.

The possibility now to revise this viewpoint and emphasise the potential impact of leadership on the quality of patient care, on service improvement and patient safety as well as organisational performance may encourage more to see leadership roles as relevant.

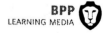

A final aspect of the CLCF that may help more clinicians into leadership roles is its foundation in a shared or distributed model of leadership and its emphasis upon leadership being integrated into the normal clinical role rather than separated from it. For many clinical staff the team leader conjures up the idea of power, position or rank of someone possessing characteristics that they simply feel they do not have. It is probably helpful then to use the term leadership rather than leader because this emphasises the point that all individual (clinicians) can make a contribution to the leadership process irrespective of their level of seniority and personal characteristics. We don't have to be something in particular to make a contribution – it can be small such as a word of advice, doing something that helps the team or ensures that an aspect of care needed by a patient is delivered when required. The behaviours described in the CLCF are accessible to all, albeit some being more easily available to some individuals than others, but all individuals can access perhaps a more limited set of leadership behaviours. In effect by each individual clinician making the leadership contribution that they can the total resource of leadership available to the organisation has increased- rather than being limited to a few senior individuals.

Chapter summary

In this chapter we learned:

- It is often the lack of good leadership skills which lead to poor patient outcomes, and breakdowns or failures in the system of care are often due to multiple factors.

- The value of leadership is further reinforced when linked to engagement and that studies have shown that in organisations which have high levels of medical engagement are usually high performing and organisations that have low levels of engagement are poor performing.

- Several studies that suggest enhanced engagement by staff in the organisation-wide goals is of benefit to the individual, as well as the organisation itself.

- It is more helpful to use the term leadership rather than leader because this emphasises the point that all individual (clinicians) can make a contribution to the leadership process irrespective of their level of seniority and personal characteristics.

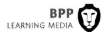

Three things to try

1. Access the latest staff or patient satisfaction, or culture survey and see how it compares with previous years.

2. Access performance data for your organisation and think about how it relates to good quality patient care.

3. Start a conversation with colleagues about the difference between positional and shared leadership.

Chapter references

Butterworth, A (2009) 'Foreword'. In Edition, Bishop, V ed. (2009) Leadership for Nursing and Allied Health Professionals: Berkshire: Open University Press.

Black, C (2008) Working for a Healthier Tomorrow: review of the health of Britain's working age population www.workingforhealth.gov.uk/documents/workingforahealthier-tomorrow

Hartley, J and Benington, J (2010) *Leadership for Healthcare*: Bristol: The Policy Press.

Lett, M The concept of clinical leadership: *Contemporary Nurse 2002; 12 (1) 16–20.*

The Mid Staffordshire NHS Foundation Trust Public Inquiry (2013) *Report of the Mid Staffordshire NHS Foundation Trust Public Inquiry, House of Commons, 2013.* London: The Stationary Office.

Macleod, D and Clarke, N (2009) Engaging for success: enhancing performance through employee engagement. *Department for Business, Innovation and Skills.*

Ovretveit, J . Leading improvement. *Journal of Health Organisation and Management. 2005; 19 (6) 413–30.*

Shipton, H, Armstrong, C, West, M, and Dawson, J. The impact of leadership and quality climate on hospital performance. *International Journal for Quality in Health Care. 2008 20 (6) 439–25*

Spurgeon, P, Clark, J, and Ham, C (2011) Medical leadership: From the dark side to centre stage. London: Radcliffe Publishing.

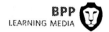

Stanley. D 'Clinical leadership and the theory of congruent leadership'. In Edition, Bishop, V ed. (2009) Leadership for Nursing and Allied Health Professionals: Berkshire: Open University Press.

Vandenberghe, C, Stordeur, S, and D'hoore, W. Transactional and transformational leadership in nursing: structural validity and substantive relationships. *European Journal of Psychological Assessment. 2002*; 18 (1) 16–29.

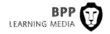

Chapter 4

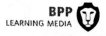

Chapter 5

Leadership, engagement and patient safety

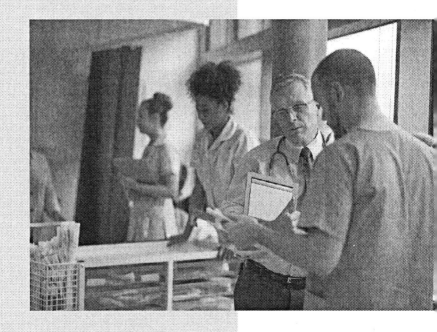

Leadership, engagement and patient safety

Chapter overview

This chapter provides:

- A description of the concepts of leadership and engagement.
- The benefits to patient safety of engaging clinicians in leadership.
- An outline of strategies to engage clinicians in leadership development.

Patient safety and clinical engagement

On February 5 2013 Robert Francis QC delivered his 2nd report of the inquiry into the Mid Staffordshire NHS Foundation Trust (Francis, 2013). This report detailed shocking accounts of failures at both an organisational and individual level that resulted in devastating consequences for the patients and their families.

The findings state that a serious failure by the Trust Board to listen sufficiently to ensure patient safety, enabled an insidious negative culture involving a tolerance of poor standards and disengagement from managerial and leadership responsibilities.

What happened in Mid Staffordshire NHS Foundation Trust was a whole range of things – from a heavy focus on targets through to not listening to patients and dismissing data. It was not one person, nor was it one group of nurses or doctors or managers. It was about allowing a culture of fear and poor style of leadership to take hold, all of which meant nurses, doctors and managers lost sight of safety and quality.

The report recommended a series of actions ranging from enforceable standards, openness, transparency and candour, improved support for care and nursing, strong patient centred healthcare leadership and accurate and useful information.

Francis specifically says that 'A leadership college should be created to provide common professional training in management and leadership' and that it 'should be a physical presence that will serve the role of reinforcing the required culture through

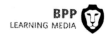

shared experience and will provide a common induction into the expectations of the NHS of those who lead and work in the system.' As described earlier the emergence of the MLCF and endorsement by the General Medical Council has seen just such provision become a normal part of medical training. The CLCF now offers the chance for all clinical professionals to access leadership training from the beginning of their career.

While not at all detracting from the seriousness of the findings of Mid Staffs inquiry, it is important to note, that the system has been working to address the issues raised for some years. Indeed the first inquiry into Mid Staffs highlighted leadership and poor quality work practices. In Chapter 2 we described the development of the CLCF and the work to embed leadership undertaken to embed the CLCF into various professional and educational standards and curricula and align with overall workforce development policy and workplace training, especially in the NHS. These initiatives were not prompted by the Francis report, but by a more general recognition of the value of clinical leadership to ensure good quality in healthcare services.

Since the establishment of the Leadership Framework (LF) tens of thousands of staff from all staff groups have taken the opportunity to assess their leadership skills with a self-assessment tool.

While impressive, these numbers are tiny when you consider the size of the NHS workforce and we contend that a broad approach is necessary to ensure the embedding of leadership behaviours into workforce development at all levels (Long & Spurgeon 2012). The full effects of this work will take time but will be more beneficial and sustainable in the longer term.

Engaging clinicians in leadership and patient safety

It is now widely held that it is vital to support patient safety by building relationships across systems of care through engaging patients, staff and boards. The most straightforward and simple definition of employee engagement is provided by MacLeod & Clarke (2009), who say it is when 'The business values the employee and the employee values the business'. They assert that the concept of engagement is a two way process involving organisations working

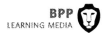

to engage employees with the latter having some degree of choice as to their response.

A single approach to both concepts has been described as engaging leadership. This is where the culture is open, accessible and transparent and when the staff member chooses whether to do the minimum, or do more (The Kings Fund, 2012).

Processes for engaging staff in leadership emphasise teamwork, collaboration and connectedness, removing barriers to communication and original thinking (The Kings Fund, 2012), and involve the persons desire to see the world through the eyes of others, to take on board their concerns and perspectives and to work with their ideas (Alimo-Metcalfe and Alban-Metcalfe, 2008). Lemer and colleagues stressed that engagement must happen at all levels of the organisation (Lemer *et al*; 2012). This theory is supported by the notion that leadership is something to be shared and used by all, but at different stages or levels.

Healthcare delivery is complex and ever-changing and, as such, requires staff exercising leadership to be able to address interconnected issues, build coalitions between disparate stakeholders, form intra- and inter-organisational partnerships and networks, and 'achieve measurable outcomes with and for communities and other stakeholders' (Bennington & Hartley, 2009). The ever-increasing need for organisations to work as part of a larger health system means that for individuals, navigating this zone of complexity requires behaviours that are adaptive. Leadership development will need to be different and utilise new methods that support and enable busy clinicians to be adaptive by 'diagnosing the system that needs to adapt to a change program, then initiating the action that needs to take place to help the system change' (Heifetz, 1995). According to Heifetz adaptive leadership is the practice of mobilising people to tackle tough challenges and thrive (Heifetz *et al*; 2009).

Clinical engagement

There has been much written on the need for clinical engagement at various levels within healthcare – at a team or service level; organisational level; professional sub-group or special interest group level (Health Workforce Australia 2011; The Kings Fund,

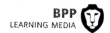

2012; The Health Foundation, 2012). From this material it is clear that 'clinical engagement' is a complex, technical, socio-political and motivational issue spanning the relevant multiple professional sub-cultures. This is underpinned by a series of inter-related factors associated with organisational context and the design of the improvement activity; and how these factors are promoted; (Parand *et al*; 2010, Spurgeon *et al*; 2011).

Where to begin the 'engagement' differs dependent on the context of the practitioner, whether student or experienced. What is clear is that the introduction to leadership concepts early in the development of all clinicians and then subsequently as their service career progresses is considered important (Long *et al*; 2012; Health and Care Professions Council, 2012; Nursing and Midwifery Council, 2010).

Without the clinical engagement at a collective level and the individual alignment of clinicians, there is no meaningful way to influence variations in practice or care (Taitz *et al*; 2011).

In 2012 the Kings Fund Commission on Leadership published a seminal work on engagement. In it they make the case for clinical engagement and provide many case studies and examples which may be of use to individuals and organisations. Engaged staff feel valued, respected and supported and through undertaking jobs with meaningful, clear tasks, some autonomy to manage their work, involvement in decision-making and supportive line managers (Kings Fund, 2012).

But engagement means far more than having an engagement strategy and approaches that lack sincerity will soon be found out because engagement is built on authenticity. Organisations that engage both staff and patients have strong values of trust, fairness and respect which are consistently articulated and acted upon (Kings Fund, 2012). It is an essential role of leadership to foster these values in their organisations.

The practical strategies for promoting and supporting clinical engagement

There is now a lot of information about strategies that promote and support clinical engagement (Spurgeon *et al*; 2011; Ham *et al*; 2013; Dickenson & Ham, 2008; Parand *et al*; 2010; Taitz *et al*; 2011). The

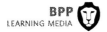

evidence regarding the impact and feasibility of various approaches is mixed and dependent on the context of the intervention and it is not realistic to expect one type of approach to solve a problem or issue (Grol, 1997).

Some of the strategies focus on the benefits, and gains, to the individual. Protecting the time doctors were allocated to spend on a program by managers was thought to be of as something that would have helped integrate doctors into the initiative (Parand *et al*; 2010).

According to Dickenson and Ham (2008), supportive organisational cultures and receptive organisational contexts are key factors.

The medical engagement tool developed by Spurgeon and colleagues, explicitly focuses on both individual and organisational conditions, expressed as 'Working in an open and fair culture', 'Having purpose and direction' and being 'Valued and empowered' (Spurgeon *et al*; 2011).

Given the multiplicity of strategies and approaches which have been shown to work and not work, a multifaceted approach would therefore seem more suited to solving a complex problem like improving health care (Grol, 1997; 2001). Braithwaite *et al* (2012) also suggest multiple interventional strategies, involving differing hierarchical levels, applying a socio-ecological logic with multiple target groups to induce systems change in inter professional collaboration.

Across the literature reviewed some practical strategies found will now be described:

Personal or individual benefit and rewards

The Health Foundation study of its quality improvement (QI) programs found that the participants' perceptions about the personal benefits obtained from the program tended to be greater than those for the organisational or service benefit (The Health Foundation, 2012). For female clinicians the benefits of involvement may be cumulative and be seen as addressing structural barriers, individual and organisational mindsets (Newman, 2011).

The use of financial and non-financial rewards is important. Clinicians and other staff want to feel valued and rewards therefore

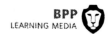

are seen as important. Rewards can come in many forms – support, time, resources, incentives, promotion, academic are some. Payment, however, is only a part and sometime not even a driver (The Health Foundation 2012; Taitz *et al*; 2011).

Engaging through personal and (inter) professional development and collaboration

Neale *et al* (2007) suggests that engagement and a change of learning and attitudes can be formulated within the training structure. Greenfield *et al* (2011) state that inter-professional learning and practice can be positively self-reinforcing and can promote improved care. However this will require changes in attitudes.

The Health Foundation (2011) found that not only do participants in their leadership program value learning together, but that they also value working alongside colleagues from different health economies.

A two-year study conducted by the Health Foundation provides a 'small but convincing case' that enabling and facilitating others to make their contribution is central to leading improvement (The Health Foundation, 2011).

Addicott *et al* (2007) found that, in a study of five cancer networks within the NHS, all but one had faced significant difficulty working together effectively, including issues such as overt and covert resistance to the concept of clinical networks, inter-professional politics, and poor communication and knowledge sharing. One characteristic of the more productive network was that it had successfully built upon pre-existing relationships that were evident before the network had been set up. Addicott *et al* also noted that the better functioning network was steered by a small group of highly motivated individuals leading them to hypothesise that this shared sense of purpose and drive played a significant role in the networks success.

Participants in quality improvement programs reviewed by The Health Foundation (2011) identified the most helpful leadership program content to be academic input, informal networking, action learning and coaching.

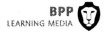

Resources

Ham (2003) states that clinicians require time to establish new practices, and recommends that managers be responsible for the provision of resources and should work closely with clinical champions. Being flexible in piloting and tailoring improvement interventions is important. Several projects in a study by The Health Foundation (2012) found it helped to take time initially to explore the improvement interventions they were offering to determine what the clinicians thought worked best.

It is crucial to provide support to maintain engagement. This includes data identification and collection, rapid and easily intelligible feedback of statistical process charts and communications to share ideas, such as newsletters and wikis (The Health Foundation, 2012). An Australian blood project successfully used social research and media to highlight a lack of congruence between prescribing patterns and best practice (Clinical Excellence Commission, 2009). A multi-channel approach was used to communicate with the target audience: the placement of print ads in relevant publications, direct marketing via personalised letters and emails signed by the campaign clinical champions, and a bespoke micro-site with an on-line debate forum and relevant resources. Additional strategies included inserting full page advertisements into the conference satchels of delegates for relevant scientific meetings, and linkages to a number of key websites. The campaign ran for a period of 15 weeks. The on-line debate was supported by an international 'virtual faculty' of transfusion experts. Over 1,700 unique visitors entered the site during the three month campaign and they spent an average five minutes reading the debates. Visitors from over 40 countries entered the site and over 60 comments were posted on the debate pages (Clinical Excellence Commission, 2009).

Managing perceptions and clear communication of the purpose

The way clinicians view a program and the manner in which it is communicated is considered to be important. Leadership behaviours have been shown to emerge when people share a common purpose (Carson *et al*; 2007). Establishing and maintaining a consistent guiding vision is viewed as important within change programs (Dickenson & Ham, 2008) and where there is a track

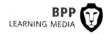

record of multiple initiatives over many years with little sign of visible commitment to on-going support, initiative overkill and decreased buy-in results (Parand *et al*; 2010).

Local program champions

The use of champions, role models and opinion leaders as agents of change is well known. The doctors' higher regard for the views of their medical peers when faced with change in their clinical practices will either facilitate or inhibit doctor engagement. This highlights the importance of selecting people for this role who have good rapport with doctors (Parand *et al*; 2010).

The use of enthusiastic individuals as a catalyst for change (such as using senior, respected and motivated professionals) and incentives (such as peer pressure and comparative audit) were also found to stimulate clinician involvement. The Health Foundation has also noted that involving the professions colleges can play a role in engaging clinicians. A later study by the Health Foundation (2012) supported the notion of influential champions further. Project champions help teams maintain engagement. Their report says that what mattered was not who the champion was, but having the right person available regularly.

Management involvement

Hamilton *et al* (2008) note the value of involving the chief executive in engagement. They recommend that chief executives seek and arrange informal opportunities for face-to-face meetings with clinical staff, play a direct role in the selection of consultants and meet newly appointed consultants, as well as attend their induction. The driver for this is that within the groups, agreement is reached on how care should be delivered to members, with emphasis being placed on achieving improvements through the intrinsic commitment of the doctors to do a good job rather than seeking compliance with targets or standards set externally (Spurgeon *et al*; 2011).

Involving service users

The involvement of service users is widely advocated and has been shown to have a powerful effect on clinicians and the way in which they view themselves and the care they provide (Coulter, 2011).

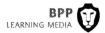

Overall, and within a range of contexts, The Health Foundation (2012) program's collective approach to service-user involvement produced positive procedural gains in individual projects and enhanced understanding among all the members of the project teams. The participants (clinicians and non-clinicians) learned the importance of understanding the different roles that various categories of service users can play, and the need to involve multiple service users on the project teams throughout their projects (The Health Foundation, 2012).

Knowledge sharing and providing opportunities for participation

There is a lot of literature and evidence about the value of regular appraisal and feedback. Taking the opportunity to feedback in different time frames. Although some learning opportunities are one-off episodes, ideally trainers should look to establish strong relationships with learners where feedback can be given, and worked on, longitudinally in time.

Conclusion

Each of these areas of activity provide an opportunity for leaders to inspire and enhance engagement in their staff and in doing so enhance safety for patients. We now turn in Chapter 6 to how educational providers, training institutions and regulators can *operate* in concert to ensure that clinicians can acquire the competencies of the CLCF in a cumulative and appropriate way to the context in which they are working.

Chapter summary

In this chapter we learned:

- The importance of leadership as a journey and something clinicians practice throughout their career.

- The concept of engagement is a two way process involving organisations working to engage employees with the latter having some degree of choice as to their response.

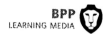

- Clinicians need to exercise leadership to be able to address interconnected issues, build coalitions between disparate stakeholders, form intra- and inter-organisational partnerships and networks, and achieve measurable outcomes with and for communities and other stakeholders.

- Without the clinical engagement at a collective level and the individual alignment of clinicians, there is no meaningful way to influence variations in practice or care.

- Practical strategies for promoting and supporting clinical engagement include Personal or individual benefit and rewards, engaging through personal and (inter) professional development and collaboration, resources, managing perceptions and clear communication of the purpose, local program champions, management involvement, involving service users, knowledge sharing and providing opportunities for participation.

 Three things to try

1. Undertake an engagement survey of staff at your organisation.

2. Think about involving local program champions in a change initiative.

3. Identify a patient advocacy group that can help you engage with colleagues.

Chapter references

Addicott, R, McGivern, G and Ferlie, E. The distortion of managerial technique? The case of clinical networks in UK healthcare. *British Journal of Management* 2007; 18, 99–105.

Alimo-Metcalfe, B Alban-Metcalfe, J (2008). Engaging Leadership: Creating organisations that maximise the potential of their people. London: Chartered Institute of Personnel and Development.

Benington, J and Hartley J (2009). Whole Systems Go! Improving Leadership Across the Whole Public Service System. Propositions to stimulate discussion and reform. London: Sunningdale Institute National School of Government.

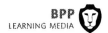

Braithwaite, J, Westbrook, M, Nugus, P, Greenfield, D, Travaglia, J, Runciman, W, Foxwell, A, R, Boyce, R,A, Devinney, T, Westbrook, J. A four-year, systems-wide intervention promoting interprofessional collaboration. *BMC Health Services Research* 2012; 12:9

Carson, J, B, Tesluk, P, E and Marone, J, A Shared leadership in teams: an investigation of antecedent conditions and performance, *Academy of Management Journal* 2007; 50, (5), 1217–1234.

Clinical Excellence Commission and National Blood Authority (2009). Evaluation Report for Blood Watch Campaign 2008. Sydney, Australia.

Coulter, A (2011). *Engaging Patients in Healthcare.* Maidenhead: Open University Press.

Dickenson, H, Ham, C (2008). Engaging doctors in leadership: Review of the literature. Jan. 2008, *Health Services Management Centre,* University of Birmingham.

Greenfield D, Nugus P, Travglia J, Braithwaite J. (2010*) Factors that shape the development of inter professional improvement initiatives in health organisations.* BMJ Quality Safety. 10. 11–36.

Grol, R. Personal Paper: Beliefs and Evidence in Changing Clinical Practice. *British Medical Journal* 1997; 315, 418–421

Grol, R. Improving the Quality of Medical Care. Building Bridges among professional pride, Payer Profit and Patient Satisfaction *Journal American Medical Association* 2001; 286, (20), 2578–2601.

Ham, C. Improving the performance of health services: the role of clinical leadership. *Lancet 2003; 361:1979–80.*

Hamilton P, Spurgeon P, Clark J, Dent J, Armit K. (2008). *Engaging doctors: can doctors influence organisational reform.* Academy of Royal Colleges & NHS Institute for Innovation and Improvement.

Health and Care Professions Council (Various) Standards of Proficiency [Online] HCPC. Available at http://www.hpc-uk.org

Health Workforce Australia (2011). *Leadership for the Sustainability of the Health System: Part 1- A Literature Review.*

Heifetz, R, Leadership Without Easy Answers. Joe Flower, a conversation with Ron Heifetz. *Healthcare Forum Journal* 1995; 38, 4.

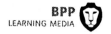

Heifetz, R, Linsky, M & Grashow, A (2009). *The practice of adaptive leadership: Tools and tactics for changing your organization and the world.* Cambridge, MA: Harvard Business Press.

Organisation and the World. (2009) Cambridge, MA, Harvard Business Press.

Lemer, C, Allwood, D, Foley, T Improving NHS Productivity: The secondary care doctors perspective. *Paper to the Kings Fund Review on leadership* 2012; London: King Fund.

Long, P,W, Spurgeon, P,C. Embedding leadership into professional, regulatory and educational standards. *International Journal of Clinical Leadership* 2012; 17, (4).

Macleod D, Clarke N. *Engaging for success: enhancing performance through employee engagement.* London. Department for Business, Innovation & Skills.

Medical Chief Executives in the NHS: Facilitators and Barriers to their Career Progress Ham, Chris and others, Health Services Management Centre for the NHS Institute for Innovation and Improvement, April 2010.

Neale G, Vincent C, Darzi A S. *The problem of engaging hospital doctors in promoting safety and quality in clinical practice J R Soc Health 2007; 127:87–94.*

Nursing and Midwifery Council (2010) Standards for pre-registration nursing education. Nursing and Midwifery Council. [Online] Available at www.standards.nmc-uk.org/PreRegNursing/Pages/Introduction.aspx [Accessed 2012].

The Health Foundation (2012). Evidence in brief: Involving primary care clinicians in quality improvement. Summary of an independent evaluation of the Engaging with Quality in Primary Care improvement programme. London: The Health Foundation.

The Kings Fund (2012). Leadership and engagement for improvement in the NHS, Together we can. *Report from The King's Fund Leadership Review, May 2012.* London: The Kings Fund.

The Mid Staffordshire NHS Foundation Trust Public Inquiry (2013) *Report of the Mid Staffordshire NHS Foundation Trust Public Inquiry, House of Commons, 2013.* London: The Stationary Office.

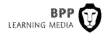

Parand, A, Burnett S, Benn J, Iskander S, Pinto A, Vincent C. Medical Engagement in organisation-wide safety and quality improvement programmes: experience in the UK Safer Patients Initiative. *Quality and Safety in Health Care* 2010; 19 (44).

Spurgeon, P, Clark, J, Ham, C (2011) *Medical Leadership: from the dark side to centre stage. London:* Radcliffe Publishing Ltd.

J. M. Taitz, T. H. Lee, and T. D. Sequist, "A Framework for Engaging Physicians in Quality and Safety," *BMJ Quality & Safety* 2011; [online].

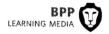

Chapter 6

The CLCF and professional, regulatory and educational standards

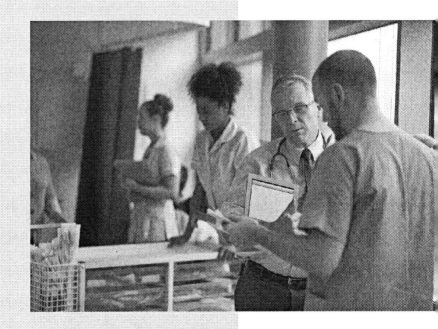

The CLCF and professional, regulatory and educational standards

Chapter overview

This chapter explores:

- The relationship between leadership and professional, regulatory and educational standards.

- Progress to embed the CLCF into higher education institutions, professional regulation, and colleges and societies.

- A case study illustrating how a clinician's practice relates to both the regulator's requirements and how the CLCF can complement and enhance the implementation of existing regulatory standards.

Introduction

There are over a million clinicians working in the UK together with another million workers, such as health care assistants and care workers, who contribute extraordinary benefit to patients and the public every day.

Approximately two thirds of these staff are highly skilled, graduate level qualified professionals and more than half of them are regulated clinical professionals, including doctors, nurses, midwives, healthcare scientists, pharmacists and a wide range of Allied Health Professionals.

All clinicians commit to a career long journey of continuous learning and development, whether refreshing or up-skilling, undertaking service improvement or research. Most of these undertake continuous professional development according to requirements set down by their professional body, such as a college or society, their employer, their registering body and higher education institutions.

The United Kingdom has one of the best health care systems in the developed world but there remains areas where we need to do much better. There continues to be failures where a lack of leadership have been identified as a significant factor.

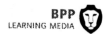

While clinicians view leadership as core to their professional value set it is not their responsibility alone to further develop the leadership capacity and capability of the workforce. They need to be supported by the system – education, professional, regulatory and employers (Long, 2011) to ensure they are able to meet the challenges of an ever changing health care system and deliver the highest possible care to people who use the services.

The purpose of this chapter is to illustrate work being undertaken to embed the CLCF into various professional and educational standards and curricula and align with overall workforce development policy and workplace training, especially in the NHS.

Workforce and system level activity

The shape and skills of the future health and public health workforce need to evolve constantly if we are to sustain high quality health services and continue to improve health in the face of demographic and technological change.

To keep up with these changes, the NHS and public health system is changing and therefore the way in which we educate and train our workforce must also change – the needs of patients and the public must be served by a workforce that has the skills and knowledge to provide safe, effective and compassionate care at all times.

Leadership development in the NHS has been underway for many years, primarily led by the NHS Institute for Innovation and Improvement (NHSI) and, since 2010, the National Leadership Council (NLC). This strategic role has recently been transferred to the NHS Leadership Academy (Academy), which was launched on the 10th April 2012. The Academy has been established to develop outstanding leadership in the health sector and take a national coordinating lead on this.

There are two other important players operating at a strategic level – Health Education England (HEE) and the Local Education and Training Boards (LETBs).

HEE will provide national leadership and oversight on strategic planning and development of the health and public health workforce, and allocate education and training resources. HEE will promote high quality education and training that is responsive to the changing

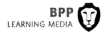

needs of patients and local communities – including responsibility for ensuring the effective delivery of important national functions, such as medical trainee recruitment.

The LETBs will be the vehicle for providers and professionals to work with HEE to improve the quality of education and training outcomes so that they meet the needs of service providers, patients and the public. Through HEE, health and public health providers will have strong input into the development of national strategies and priorities so education and training can adapt quickly to new ways of working and new models of service. LETBs may also take on specific leadership roles for particular professional groups, such as the smaller professions and commissioning specialist skills.

Education Outcomes Framework

The Education Outcomes Framework (EOF) will set expectations across the whole education and training system so that investment in developing the health and public health workforce supports the delivery of excellent healthcare and health improvement. LETBs and HEE will use the Education Outcomes Framework as the basis for developing the operating model and working arrangements with partners (Department of Health, 2012).

Leadership behaviours are inherent within the EOF (see EOF outcomes below):

1. **Excellent education** – Education and training is commissioned and provided to the highest standards, ensuring learners have an excellent experience and that all elements of education and training are delivered in a safe environment for patients, staff and learners.

2. **Competent and capable staff** – There are sufficient health staff educated and trained, aligned to service and changing care needs, to ensure that people are cared for by staff who are properly inducted, trained and qualified, who have the required knowledge and skills to do the jobs the service needs, whilst working effectively in a team.

3. **Adaptable and flexible workforce** – The workforce is educated to be responsive to changing service models and responsive to innovation and new technologies with knowledge about best practice, research and innovation, that promotes adoption and dissemination of better quality service delivery to reduces variability and poor practice.

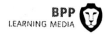

4. **NHS values and behaviours** – Healthcare staff have the necessary compassion, values and behaviours to provide person centred care and enhance the quality of the patient experience through education, training and regular Continuing Personal and Professional Development (CPPD) that instils respect for patients.

5. **Widening participation** – Talent and leadership flourishes free from discrimination with fair opportunities to progress and everyone can participate to fulfil their potential, recognising individual as well as group differences, treating people as individuals, and placing positive value on diversity in the workforce and there are opportunities to progress across the five leadership framework domains.

Embedding the CLCF into professional, regulatory & educational standards

The CLCF is applicable across the UK as clinicians' train and work in many settings and sectors across the four home countries. It is designed to be used in conjunction with the relevant professional and service documents provided by the professional bodies, government bodies, regulators and higher education institutions (see Figure 6.1).

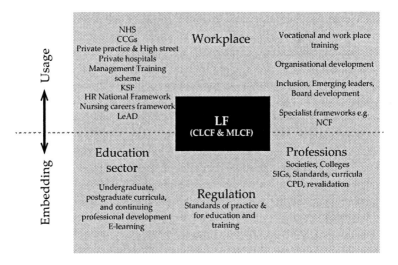

Figure 6.1 Relationship between CLCF and standards

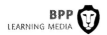

Professions (colleges and societies)

Although not all clinicians necessarily belong to a professional body, most of the clinical professions are nonetheless, represented by a college, society or association. These organisations play an important role in setting standards and representing the interests of their discipline in important debates. Many of these have now begun to recognise the importance of leadership and that it is something that is nested in their own professional values and belief structures (Long *et al*; 2011).

The professional bodies are at different stages in adopting the CLCF and several of the large professions have undertaken work to adopt the CLCF.

The British Psychological Society (BPS) has published a Clinical Psychology Leadership Development Framework and is now actively planning on similar extension into other areas of practice, such as occupational psychology. The BPS Learning Centre is designing a new leadership course and undertaking a review of its product offerings in relation to the CLCF.

The Royal Pharmaceutical Society has published its own highly contextualised version of the CLCF Royal Pharmaceutical Society (2011). The Centre for Postgraduate Pharmacy Education (CPPE) now has a learning module for pharmacists. The Supporting Leadership Series 19 has been designed around the CLCF domains with a launch event, pre and post activities and a series of self-directed modules run over a 12 month period (Centre for Postgraduate Pharmacy Education, 2012a & 2012b).

Within the nursing profession there is a significant drive to further develop leadership capability although much has already been done. The Royal College of Nursing (RCN) which has commenced developing a highly contextualised CLCF for nursing and has identified some exciting possibilities for dissemination via their CPD learning zone.

The Chief Scientist is supporting the development of a national programme that uses the CLCF as a basis for structuring healthcare science leadership and integrating it into other professions and across healthcare organisations.

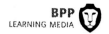

The Society and College of Radiography will be reviewing its Learning Development Framework in 2012 and will be extending this to cover all areas of practice. They intend to shape this work around the CLCF.

The College of Operating Department Practitioners (CODP) has enhanced their curriculum guidance, which was published in the early 2011 to better reflect the need for leadership and relate the competencies to the CLCF.

The British Dietetic Association has begun to introduce the CLCF to its members along with links through to the NHS Leadership Academy website and other related material.

Regulation

An important link to embedding leadership behaviours into the clinical professions is through regulatory standards (Long *et al*; 2013). Behaviours that all clinicians must demonstrate are described in the various policy, guidance, standards of proficiency, standards of education, codes of conduct and ethical behaviour set down by the professions' regulators, which are intended to assure the safety of those using the services and the public generally. Each of these bodies maintains and publishes a register of practitioners that meet these standards and are legally able to practise in the United Kingdom:

- Health and Care Professions Council (HCPC)
- Nursing and Midwifery Council (NMC)
- General Optical Council (GOC)
- General Dental Council (GDC)
- General Pharmaceutical Council (GPhC)
- General Medical Council (GMC)
- General Osteopathic Council (GOsC)
- General Chiropractic Council (GCC)

Clinicians may wonder why they must meet the requirements set down by their regulator and also undertake additional development related to the leadership.

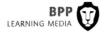

The primary focus of regulation for registered clinicians is on their 'professional' practice but unfortunately, there is little hard evidence around how professional regulation impacts on the behaviours of the individual practitioner and fitness to practice proceedings are rarely about technical competence (Council for Healthcare Regulatory Excellence, 2011; NHS Leadership Academy, 2011). However, all clinicians work in systems and most within organisations and the CLCF describes these 'professional' behaviours and combines them with behaviours designed to make staff operate with a great awareness of the system, their role in it and how to take action, influence change, and drive innovation and improvement.

The following case study illustrates how a clinician's practice relates to both her regulator's requirements and how the CLCF can complement and enhance the implementation of existing regulatory standards.

Case Study 1

The following illustrates the applicable Domains, Elements and respective competency statements from the CLCF and how these can link in with the clinician's own professional standards.

Anne is an occupational therapist working in an acute mental health setting where patients (service users) have been detained under section three of the mental health act 1983 and are therefore unable to leave the hospital. She became aware of a need for patients to have a designated space within the confines of the hospital where they could carry out some therapeutic outdoor activity.

She was already working to the Health and Care Professions Council's standards of proficiency (abbreviated henceforth to HCPC SoP) for occupational therapists and used her professional body's post qualifying framework to plan her longer term career development. When she became aware of the CLCF, she decided to incorporate this as a further tool to inform her plans and monitor her progress.

Several service users had mentioned to her that they had no opportunity for fresh air and physical exercise that was also productive. She identified an unmet need and set about planning a service development that would meet patients' requirements. Anne recognised the need for patients to be fully provided for even though, or especially because, they were confined (CLCF Domain 1 Demonstrating Personal Qualities, Element (iv) Acting with Integrity). Communicating effectively with individuals, appreciating their social, cultural, religious and ethnic backgrounds and their age, gender and abilities; valuing, respecting and promoting equality and diversity). She

---

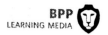

reflected on the value of a horticultural group for patients who could then have access to meaningful activity. She researched the efficacy of a horticultural group in promoting well-being and recovery (HPC SoP 2b: formulation and delivery of plans and strategies for meeting health and social care needs; 2b.1 to be able to use research, reasoning and problem-solving skills to determine appropriate actions; CLCF Domain 4 Improving Services, Element 4(iii) Encouraging Improvement: question the status quo; act as positive role model for innovation; encourage dialogue and debate with a wide range of people; develop creative solutions to transform services and care).

She carried out a risk assessment (HPC Sof P 3a.3 understand the need to establish and maintain a safe practice environment; CLCF Domain 4 Improving services, Element 4(i) Ensuring Patient Safety; identify and quantify the risk to patients using information from a range of sources; use evidence, both positive and negative, to identify options; use systematic ways of assessing and minimising risk).

She found a piece of unused waste ground within the boundaries of the hospital. (CLCF Domain 3 Managing Services, Element 3(ii) Managing resources – minimise waste). She recruited colleagues and prepared a business case to convince her superiors of the worth of this project (HPC SoP1b Professional relationships, 1b.1 be able to work, where appropriate, in partnership with other professionals, support staff, service users and their relatives and carers; CLCF Domain 2 Working with others, Element 2(iv) Working within teams – willing to lead a team, involving the right people at the right time CLCF Domain 3 Element 3(i) Planning – gather feedback from patients, service users and colleagues to help develop plans). She drew on her reflective log to write up the project for her professional magazine in order that peers might adapt her approach for their own workplace settings (HPC SoP 2c.2 be able to audit, reflect on and review practice – understand the value of reflection on practice and the need to record the outcome of such reflection (CLCF Domain 5 Setting direction, Element 5(iv) Evaluating Impact – formally and informally disseminate good practice).

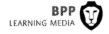

All the key bodies responsible for professional regulation are exploring how to approach leadership and they are at various stages of adoption and coverage within their pre- and post-registration approaches.

- **The General Medical Council** has embedded the medical leadership competencies in the standards for undergraduate medical education and training and has approved postgraduate specialty curricula for all the Medical Royal Colleges and Faculties that integrate the competencies. The competencies are also covered in new guidance for all doctors on leadership and management responsibilities published in January 2012.

- **The Nursing and Midwifery Council** (2010) has recently published its standards for pre-registration nursing education and there is excellent coverage of leadership. There is an opportunity to embed leadership in practice through the review of the standards of conduct, performance and ethics for nurses and midwives.

- **The Health and Care Professions Council (HCPC)** is supportive of the CLCF. The HCPC is currently reviewing the standards of proficiency for the professions it regulates. After revising the generic standards of proficiency that apply to all HCPC registrants, the HCPC Council decided not to include a standard on leadership in the generic standards. However, the issue of leadership will be considered in the profession specific standards. As part of the ongoing review of the standards of proficiency, each profession will be able to recommend whether relevant leadership requirements should be included in the profession specific standards for their profession. The standards of proficiency are used by education providers to set curricula for pre-registration education and training in higher education institutions that provide training for the professions regulated by the HCPC and in September 2012 the HCPC published a paper setting out its position on the CLCF and what it might mean to education providers (HCPC, 2012).

- **The General Dental Council** has recently published a learning outcomes framework to replace the existing curricula for all the registration categories. Management and leadership is one of the four domains providing the structure to the new outcomes. There is excellent coverage across all the domains of the CLCF. This is intended to provide a continuum with education and post- registration practise. The GDC is also

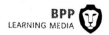

currently developing a revalidation policy and process, and the domains here reflect the same structure. Again, one of the domains is management and leadership and this should provide the opportunity to influence the continuing practice leadership competences.

- The newly established **General Pharmaceutical Council (GPhC)** has identified leadership issues as ones they want to work on further, and will shortly be establishing a group to consider whether there is scope for further enhancement of leadership coverage in GPhC education and training standards. Leadership is a hot topic in pharmacy regulation, particularly following the introduction of compulsory registration of pharmacy technicians. The plan is to develop additional regulatory guidance on team working in pharmacy, which will include significant leadership coverage on the shared leadership model, as well as exploring positional leadership issues relevant to the complexity and diversity of pharmacy practice. These issues will also be considered in the context of GPhC work to develop new standards for retail pharmacy business at registered pharmacies.

- **The General Optical Council (GOC)** is reviewing its standards of competence to integrate the CLCF and we are providing input to the review. The GOC is planning on strengthening the statement within its Code of Conduct.

- **The General Osteopathy Council (GosC)** has a number of routes available for describing leadership in osteopathy regulation. These include compulsory CPD scheme, standards of training and re-validation standards/criteria. The GosC will need to lead and inform pre-registration documentation, though they have indicated this could take some time.

- **The General Chiropractic Council (GCC)** reviews its Code of Practice and Standard of Proficiency (COP & SOP) approximately every five years. The last review took place between 2008 and 2009 and the revised COP & SOP was published with an implementation date from 30 June 2010. The GCC's Degree Recognition Criteria (the outcomes and standards that pre-registration chiropractic programmes have to meet for access to the profession) are based on the COP & SOP. The Degree Recognition Criteria were reviewed following the COP & SOP review and published in 2010.

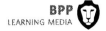

Higher Education

Ensuring that clinical staff are introduced to management or leadership concepts early in their educational development and then subsequently as their service career progresses is important. Not only does this parallel successful models but it also captures the widespread viewpoint that early introduction normalises the material such that clinical professionals are encouraged to see such activities as an inherent part of their role, rather than something to which they are introduced later in their careers (Long & Spurgeon, 2012).

Many Higher Education Institutions (HEIs) are involved in provision of pre- and post-registration education to clinicians. Unlike in medicine, which is very structured across the specialties, approaching this task for the non-medical clinical professions is more complicated because:

- There are many more professional groups and regulatory bodies.
- Different education models across the groups – a simple concept of undergraduate provision is replaced by pre-registration and post-registration courses of similar but not precise equivalence.
- Different timescales to the training routes.
- Limited regulation of the post-registration training content.

For example, in pre-registration education, there are over 1,000 courses across almost 200 providers in the UK. For post registration education, there are over 150 courses across 30 providers (not including CPD-specific or research-based degrees).

Pre-registration education routes vary by profession. For example:

- Some train via vocational training (operating department practitioners, paramedics).
- Many require specific undergraduate degrees (optometrists, midwives, nurses, speech and language therapists etc).
- Others proceed through relevant undergraduate and postgraduate degrees to further training (doctors, psychologists, pharmacists).
- Some require relevant postgraduate degrees but do not have specific undergraduate requirements (music therapists).

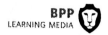

There is a critical link between regulation and education & training. Though there is little evidence of the effects of health care professional regulation on those regulated, describing leadership behaviours in regulatory standards at all stages is vital because of the importance placed on it in assuring the quality of standards of practice and care delivered to patients. It is also important because HEIs relate their content to the minimum standards set down by the relevant regulators (Long & Spurgeon, 2012).

More than any other activity, describing leadership in regulation will drive changes to education and training and this will eventually lead to an increase in the leadership capability within the system (Long *et al*; 2011; Long & Spurgeon, 2012).

Preceptorship programmes

Many health practitioners across a wide range of organisations already benefit from well-established preceptorship schemes. This foundation period for practitioners at the start of their careers helps them begin the journey from novice to expert and is an ideal stage to set out the range of leadership behaviours that all clinicians are expected to be able to demonstrate across all five domains of the CLCF.

There are plans to develop a national programme for all newly qualified nurses, midwives and allied health professionals in NHS England. This programme will be designed to support the transition from student to newly qualified health professional by supporting learning in everyday practice through a range of learning activities. There is a clear link to the CLCF and it would be positive development to see the programme extended to support career progression and transition over a more extended timeframe.

Chapter summary

In this chapter we have learned:

- The relationship between leadership behaviours and professional standards.

- Introducing leadership concepts early in the development of all clinicians and then subsequently as their service career progresses is important.

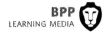

- While clinicians view leadership as core to their professional value set it is not their responsibility alone to further develop the leadership capacity and capability of the workforce. They need to be supported by the system – education, professional, regulatory and employers.

- Describing leadership in professional regulation will drive changes to education and training and this will eventually lead to an increase in the leadership capability within the system.

 Three things to try

1. Develop and implement a learning plan for an identified practice development.

2. Ask colleagues whether they'd like to set up a team development activity.

3. Think about your own leadership practice and ask colleagues how this experience compares with their own.

Chapter references

A scoping study on the effects of health professional regulation on those regulated (2011) Unpublished Final report submitted to the Council for Healthcare Regulatory Excellence.

Centre for Postgraduate Pharmacy Education (2012). Developing Pharmacy Leadership Series. *School of Pharmacy and Pharmaceutical Sciences*, University of Manchester.

Centre for Postgraduate Pharmacy Education (2012). Inspiring future Pharmacy Leadership Series. *School of Pharmacy and Pharmaceutical Sciences*, University of Manchester.

Department of Health (2012) Liberating the NHS: Developing the Healthcare Workforce from Design to Delivery. London: Gateway Reference 16977.

Health Care Professions Council (2012) HCPC Position Statement on NHS Clinical Leadership Competency Framework. HCPC. [Online] Available at HYPERLINK "http://www.hpc-uk.org/assets/documents/10003C4404-positionstatementonleadership.pdf"www.hpc-uk.org/assets/documents/10003C4404-positionstatementonleadership.pdf .

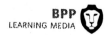

Long, P, W et al. The CLCF: developing leadership capacity and capability in the clinical professions. *International Journal of Clinical Leadership 2011; 17 No. 2*

Long P,W, Spurgeon, P, C. Embedding leadership into professional, regulatory and educational standards. *International Journal of Clinical Leadership 2012; 17, (4).*

Long, P W et al (2013) The challenge of leadership education in primary care in the UK. *Education for Primary Care Winter Special Edition 2013; 24, (1).*

NHS Leadership Academy (2011) Embedding leadership into professional regulation, London.

Royal Pharmaceutical Society (2011) Leadership competency Framework for pharmacy professionals. *Royal Pharmaceutical Society*, London.

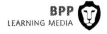

Chapter 6

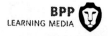

Chapter 7

Leadership learning at pre-qualifying stage

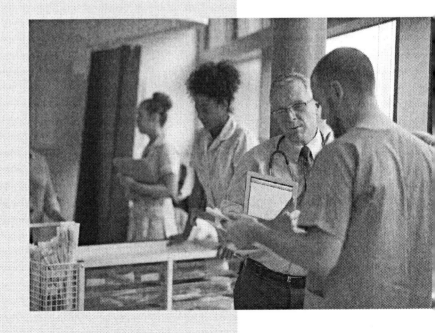

Leadership learning at pre-qualifying stage

Chapter overview

This chapter explores:

- Pre-qualification training and how it relates to the five domains of the CLCF.

- A description of how to exercise leadership on clinical placements and when working within teams.

- Three case studies describing leadership in practice.

Introduction

As an undergraduate or in training to be a clinician there is an array of knowledge and skills to be learned, not least of these skills is learning to be a leader. Good clinical leadership is seen as key to maintaining patient safety and improving patient experience.

Learning about leadership should be central to personal development and this learning should be supported by your accredited university programme. Indeed, it is now a mandatory requirement for pre-registration education and training for nurses to include leadership and the Health Care Professions Council is also supportive of the CLCF. Many higher education institutions are now beginning to introduce leadership into the undergraduate curriculum. For example, the Faculty of Health and Social Care of the University of Chester now introduces the concept of leadership to first year nursing students using the CLCF self-assessment tool as part of the 'Learning to be a Professional' module. Students are introduced to reflection, self-assessment, and the use of differing frameworks as guidance to personal, professional and service development. As part of this process, students undertake the CLCF self-assessment tool, initially focusing on Domains One and Two (Demonstrating Personal Qualities and Working with Others respectively) as a starting point for development of both reflective and leadership skills, before using the tool to review other domains to evidence an emerging level of competence once practice learning experience has begun. This self-assessment is then discussed and banked in

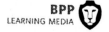

the student's portfolio within the practice learning module and a formative action plan for key points developed within the students' portfolio (see Case Study 3 later in this chapter).

Initially identifying opportunities to develop leadership and management skills may be challenging, however there will be numerous opportunities some obvious and some you will need to seek out. Taking opportunities to improve care for patients can enrich placement experience and integrate individuals into the clinical team more effectively. Opportunities can vary significantly and may be small scale; identifying areas for change such as improving patient information leaflets or becoming engaged in larger scale projects already underway in the placement area as many services are undergoing a period of change.

Undergraduates may have more time to communicate with patients, this shouldn't be a wasted opportunity. Understanding the patient's experience and their perception of the care being provided can give valuable insight in to how care can be improved; individuals may find they are able to give a different perspective on an issue or situation as they are not constrained by established ways of doing things.

The domains of the framework are underpinned by the professions respective codes of conduct (Nursing and Midwifery Council, 2010 and Health and Care Professions Council, 2008) and should be read in conjunction with the respective code.

CLCF Domains

Demonstrating Personal Qualities

As part of personal development students should explore areas such as self-awareness and how their beliefs, attitudes and actions can impact upon not only their learning and development but also patient care. Revelations regarding the poor care and treatment of patients have damaged the reputation of the NHS over recent years. Treating patients as people can improve the quality of care. This is particularly pertinent in the care of the elderly and particular approaches to care such as the person-centred framework (McCormack & McCance, 2010) and the biographical approach (Clarke *et al*; 2003) have been developed specifically to improve attitudes to hospitalised older patients.

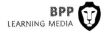

Working with Others

Patient safety and quality of care relies heavily on good communication and team work (Leonard *et al*; 2004), working well in a multi professional team is imperative and students need to explore their attitudes and behaviours to ensure effective integration into clinical teams on placement. Poorly organised and dysfunctional teams can have an adverse effect on the patient experience. As a student understanding what makes a good team, and their responsibility in enhancing that team is crucial to every placement experience. Take for example, a case study of a student who finds himself in the middle of a peer discussion about the ethics of funding breast cancer patients with high-cost drugs. The group members are all expressing views at the same time and talking over their colleagues. He notices that one member of the group has become visibly distressed, and is about to leave the room. He asks the group to pause, and suggests a break for coffee. He then speaks to the distressed student to check that she is able to continue as he feels that the discussion may be creating distress about a recent family bereavement. When the group resumes, he suggests ways in which they could improve their discussions by listening and taking turns to speak.

Managing Services

Organisations are under extreme pressure to function efficiently and effectively within constrained budgets and resources. Students will not take a lead in managing services; however in preparation for their future career it is vital they develop an understanding of resource allocation to ensure they develop the knowledge and skills to manage and deploy resources effectively in the future. Understanding how NHS services are planned, funded and evaluated is crucial to the future success of the NHS.

Improving Services

Healthcare is a dynamic environment with services evolving in light of new evidence. Improving services for the benefit of patients is an ongoing process. Students can take responsibility for simple but effective interventions such has ensuring patient observation charts are completed accurately and in a timely manner and fluid charts are accurate, these actions can minimise risk to patients.

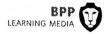

Various methodologies have been adopted by the NHS to support ongoing service improvement. One of these is PDSA (Plan Do Study Act) cycle which provides the framework for continuous improvement.

The four stages of the PDSA cycle:

1. PLAN – the change to be tested or implemented.

2. DO – carry out the test or change.

3. STUDY – data before and after change and reflect on what was learned.

4. ACT – plan the next change cycle or full implementation.

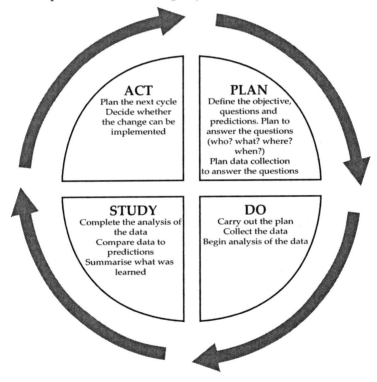

Figure 7.1 PDSA Model (Source: NHS Institute for Innovation and Improvement)

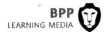

Improving patient experience

There is a growing recognition that patient experience directly affects outcomes (Little *et al*; 2001), interacting and communicating with patients are essential to improving their experience of the healthcare system. Undergraduates will have time to develop a rapport with patients, seeking to understand their experiences and perceptions as they journey through the system.

Setting Direction

As an undergraduate your exposure to the wider operational context of the NHS is limited, however developing your understanding of the key policies shaping the NHS is central to their knowledge and understanding of the wider influences on healthcare. Healthcare is a dynamic environment with regular changes to policy effecting how patients access services such as care closer to home, patient choice, National Institute for Clinical Excellence (NICE) guidance, changes to commissioning and financial processes. Developing an understanding about how and why decisions are made will enhance their knowledge and prepare them for challenges which lie ahead in their professional career.

The following three case studies provide examples of how individuals have used and integrated acquisition of leadership skills in the CLCF with their learning about clinical practice. It is clear that each case study makes use of a number of different leadership skills within the CLCF. This is true of all skilled, complex behaviour. It is rare that just one competence alone is at work. The seamless integration of these skills is effectively leadership in operation. The reader may find a copy of the CLCF useful to have alongside whilst using the case studies.

Case Study 1 Improving services within the team

While a student at university, Alexia undertook a service improvement project on the resuscitation process within the Accident and Emergency department in a hospital trust. During the project Alexia referred to the CLCF to help inform her actions and decisions. The following case study illustrates how clinical leadership can be demonstrated by a student with reference to CLCF elements. The case study demonstrates that Alexia's work shows leadership particularly in the: Domain 2 Working with Others, Domain 4 Improving Services and Domain 5 Setting Direction.

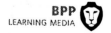

Alexia found that at the time there were was no nationally available statistical data regarding the number of cardiac arrests, and little available benchmark data (Domain 5 Setting Direction, Element 5(i) Identifying the context for change). In her own hospital there was on average one cardiac arrest a day and Alexia set out to investigate what happened when cardiac arrests occurred, and how the response could be improved (Domain 5 Setting Direction, Element 5(ii) Applying knowledge and evidence). She used a process mapping tool, walking through patients' journeys and listening to patients' stories to identify areas that could be improved. As a result she identified four parts of the process which could be improved (Domain 4 Improving Services, Element 4(ii) Critically evaluating).

From this analysis, Alexia identified one area which she considered most critical in terms of enhancing patient safety.

This related to the restocking of the resuscitation trolley. There had been a checklist for what equipment should be on the trolley but this did not always correlate with what was actually on the trolley. This could potentially result in a patient being harmed or dying should an item be missing. Alexia wanted to develop a system whereby, whatever the staff member's level of experience, they would easily and safely be able to re-stock the trolley such that the correct items would be available on the next occasion of use (Domain 4 Improving Services, Element 4(i) Ensuring patient safety).

For her improvement project, Alexia created and piloted a bespoke checklist in line with current DH resuscitation policy that would allow staff of all levels of experience to follow and complete. It encompassed all the correct equipment and drugs on the list, in the correct location within the trolley. She recognised that to implement such a change effectively she would need to engage staff so they would support and welcome the change (Domain 2 Working With Others, Element 2(iii) Encouraging contribution). She recognised the importance of communication and training to ensure that all relevant staff restocked the trolley according to the list, otherwise the chain would be broken (Domain 3 Managing Services, Element 3(iii) Managing people).

In implementing the change, Alexia used the PDSA cycle. Planning involved working with others in planning the trial and benchmarking against other trusts (Domain 2 Working With Others, Element 2(iii) Encouraging contribution, Domain 4 Improving Services, Element 4(iii) Encouraging improvement). Doing was a weeklong pilot with daily feedback from staff using the new and old checklists (Domain 5 Setting Direction, Element 5(ii) Applying knowledge and evidence). Studying involved analysing the results and determining any modifications (Domain 5 Setting Direction, Element 5(iii) Making decisions). Acting involved extending the trial and reporting findings of the project to the hospital's resuscitation committee (Domain 5 Setting Direction, Element 5(iv) Evaluating impact).

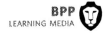

Alexia knew that sustaining the change would be critical and that strong leadership would be important. She identified potential obstacles to successful implementation and put in place mechanisms to ensure long term success, such as assigning someone responsible for keeping the checklist up to date, and making the checklist easily available on the intranet (Domain 4 Improving Services, Element 4(iv) Innovation and facilitating transformation). The checklist is now being updated and used within the trust, and all trolleys in the trust are being changed in accordance with a common list, increasing standardisation and further enhancing patient safety.

Alexia reflected on her personal learning throughout the process and was an active member of an action learning set (Domain 1 Demonstrating Personal Qualities, Element 1(iii) Continuing professional development). Key learning points for her were: recognising the value of different perspectives (Domain 2 Working With Others, Element 2(ii) Building and maintaining relationships); appreciating that change cannot be made by a single person and relies on teamwork and collaboration (Domain 2 Working With Others, Element 2(iv) Working within teams); the importance of developing networks within and external to any organisation in order to achieve sustained patient safety improvement (Domain 2 Working With Others, Element 2(i) Developing networks). She was successful in negotiating a week's work experience at John Hopkins hospital in the USA where she learned about their approach to resuscitation. This provided her with further ideas for how to improve the resuscitation process in future.

Alexia used the CLCF self-assessment tool which she found useful in understanding her development needs and determining a personal development plan.

Case Study 2 Exploring the patient/clinician relationship

During a clinical placement in the community setting, Naomi conducted a booking appointment with a primigravid woman (first pregnancy). At the appointment, the woman stated that she would like a homebirth. On further discussions it became apparent that she had several risk factors which would usually exclude her from delivering at home, due to the danger these risks factors pose. Despite informing the woman of these risks and explaining that the preferred place of birth would be the hospital, she insisted on having a homebirth. In this case, Naomi used the CLCF to guide her decision making and actions, showing that leadership qualities can and need to be developed and demonstrated as a student midwife. All domains of the CLCF were used, but particularly Domain 1 (Demonstrating Personal Qualities), Domain 2 (Working with Others), Domain 3 (Managing Services) and Domain 4 (Improving Services).

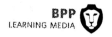

The Demonstrating Personal Qualities domain was utilised in several ways. Firstly, Naomi developed self-awareness (Element 1(i) Developing self-awareness) by considering her own personal and professional values in relation to the woman's wishes. She recognised that conflict could arise as her personal opinions differed from her patient's, and ensured that she did not let this affect her judgement or care (Element 1(iv) Acting with integrity). Secondly, Naomi identified that her knowledge in some area's relating to the case were lacking, and so took the opportunity to further her learning to ensure that she could provide better care and leadership (Element 1(iii) Continuing Professional Development). For example, the woman was affected by genital herpes, and so Naomi researched the condition further to identify how this could affect pregnancy and childbirth, and how the risk of transmission to the child could be reduced. Naomi also reflected on her actions by using Gibb's (1998) reflective cycle considering what happened, her thoughts and feelings and an evaluation, conclusion and action plan. This aided Naomi's professional development and prepared her for a similar situation were it to occur in the future.

Elements from the domain 'Working with Others' were also referred to. A trusting and supportive relationship was built between the woman and the healthcare team to ensure that a suitable plan of care was made and followed (Element 2(ii) Building and maintain relationships). An equal partnership was developed in which the woman was encouraged to involve herself in the decision-making, following the Royal College of Obstetricians and Gynaecologist's recommendation that women with recurrent genital herpes should have an individualised management plan regarding mode of delivery (RCOG, 2007). This relationship was maintained by effective communication, and showing understanding of the woman's wishes and the healthcare professionals' concerns.

Furthermore, Naomi arranged for the woman to discuss her situation with a consultant midwife who specialised in homebirths, demonstrating that she was aware of and used the networks and services that were available to her (Element 2(i) Developing networks). Naomi also actively encouraged discussion of the case within the community team with which she was working, seeking their opinions on the decision-making process (Element 2(iii) Encouraging contribution). This not only supported Naomi in her role, but also helped develop and educate the other members of the team. A Supervisor of Midwives was also involved to support Naomi and the midwives to practice safely and effectively, whilst being an advocate for the woman (Duerden, 2009; NMC, 2004).

Naomi contributed to Managing Services by assisting in planning the care and services that were to be given to the woman. Different options were considered, including allowing the woman to have her baby on a low risk unit,

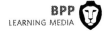

and the risks and benefits were discussed (Element 3(i) Planning). Once a plan was put in place, Naomi helped to gather the necessary resources in order to deliver safe care (Element 3(ii) Managing resources). For example, she prepared the homebirth box that was to be delivered to the woman's house several weeks before her due date, using a checklist to make sure that all the appropriate and necessary equipment was present and alerting her mentor to any items that were missing. Naomi sought the woman's feedback on the care planning process and used this to inform future planning (Element 3(i) Planning).

The CLCF domain Improving Services was also used by Naomi in this case. Naomi contributed to a risk assessment, in which the risks specific to the woman were systematically identified and critically assessed. Once these had been highlighted they were responded to by putting steps into place to minimise the risks (Element 4(i) Ensuring patient safety). For example, a plan was made for transfer to hospital, should an emergency situation arise. In order to further assist in improving the service offered by the community midwives for homebirths, Naomi critically evaluated the care that had been offered to the woman, how the risks were managed and the outcome (Element 4(ii) Critically evaluates). The woman went into labour at night, and due to low staffing levels on the night shift there was not a midwife available to attend her at home, and she was asked to go into hospital. Naomi discussed this issue with the team and ways to reorganise the distribution of staff were considered, such as having an on call community midwife every night.

The term 'leader' does not immediately come to mind when considering the role of a student midwife, but this case clearly shows that leadership qualities can and should be developed during undergraduate training. The CLCF demonstrates the responsibility that student midwives have to develop skills of leadership to enhance the quality of care for patients. By working within the domains of the CLCF, student midwives can have a significant impact on women's experiences and contribute to the standard of leadership within the service provided.

Case Study 3 Introducing leadership to the undergraduate curriculum

The Faculty of Health and Social Care of the University of Chester views the CLCF as a key resource thread throughout the programme to enable students to meet the learning outcomes of the various modules. They have identified the links between module content and the elements of the CLCF.

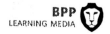

In year one, within the Learning to be a Professional module, the concept of leadership and the leadership framework is introduced. Students are introduced to reflection, self- assessment, and the use of differing frameworks as guidance to personal, professional and service development. As part of this process, students undertake the CLCF self-assessment tool, initially focussing on Domains One and Two (Demonstrating Personal Qualities and Working with Others respectively) as a starting point for development of both reflective and leadership skills, before using the tool to review other domains to evidence an emerging level of competence once practice learning experience has begun.

This self-assessment is then discussed and banked in the student's portfolio within the practice learning module and a formative action plan for key points developed within the student's portfolio.

Within the second clinical placement, students again use the CLCF self-assessment tool to review their behaviour with regard to CLCF Domains Three and Four (Managing Services and Improving Services respectively) during clinical simulation and debriefing session.

Within the module The Determinants of Health and Wellbeing, Domains One and Two are again considered, along with domain three in relation to contributing to planning service delivery and managing risk.

In year two the module Practice Learning Two continues to use the CLCF as a means of examining leadership behaviours in both the students themselves, and the clinical staff they are observing and working alongside. The concept of self-assessment is then further discussed and banked in the student's portfolio within the practice learning module and the formative action plans updated within the student's portfolio.

Within the module, The Value of Evidence in Professional Practice, the service improvement and change management aspects of the CLCF are focussed upon. At this point elements from Domain Five (Setting Direction) are introduced and considered alongside Domains One to Four.

One of the learning outcomes in the module Field Specific Nursing Practice specifically focuses on collaborative working with healthcare professionals and service users and again draws upon themes based within the CLCF when learning within field specific sessions.

The module Preparing for Future Practice is a key leadership and management module within the programme. It encourages students to reflect on their learning prior to registration and provides a vehicle for planning future professional development. The CLCF again maps directly to the module learning outcomes, and is particularly useful in focusing on supporting other healthcare workers and the learning environment in the future.

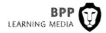

In year three the Practice Learning Three module, draws all five CLCF domains together, and the self-assessment tool is again used to clarify personal development and prepare an action plan for future preceptorship. At the completion of this module, it is anticipated that all components of the CLCF domains are evidenced.

The module Co-ordinating Complexities in Care Delivery further develops the student's ability and knowledge when managing case loads and working collaboratively as a nurse leader.

The Critical Perspectives in Health and Social Care module again draws learning from all five domains of the CLCF together with a particular focus on service design and delivery, whilst allowing the student to experience setting direction through enterprise and initiative.

The CLCF domain structure will be an appendix within the Clinical Skills Inventory to allow for ease of cross referencing when in practice and form a structured part of the student's electronic portfolio.

Chapter summary

In this chapter we learned:

- A clinician's leadership journey begins in their pre-qualifying training and continues throughout their career.

- Learning about leadership should be central to an individual's personal development and this learning should be supported by their accredited university programme.

- Many higher education institutions are now beginning to introduce leadership into the undergraduate curriculum.

- There are many opportunities for students to exercise leadership such as clinical placements.

Three things to try

1. Complete the CLCF self-assessment http://www.leadershipacademy. nhs.uk/wp-content/uploads/2012/11/NHSLeadership-Framework-CLCFSelfAssessmentTool.pdf

2. Reflect on the results and what your strengths and weaknesses are.

3. Share what you have learned with colleagues during end of term discussions.

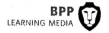

Chapter references

Clarke A, Hanson E, J and Ross, H Seeing the person behind the patient: enhancing the care of older people using a biographical approach. *Journal of Clinical Nursing*; 2003; 12: 697–706.

Duerden J (2009). Midwifery supervision and clinical governance. In: FRASER, D.M., COOPER, MA (eds) Myles Textbook for Midwives. 15th edition. Oxford: Churchill Livingstone. 999–1014.

Gibbs G (1988). Learning by Doing: A guide to teaching and learning methods. *Further Education Unit*. Oxford Polytechnic: Oxford.

Health and Care Professions Council (Various) Standards of Proficiency [Online] HCPC. Available at http://www.hpc-uk.org

Health and Care Professions Council (2008) Standards of conduct, performance and ethics [Online] HCPC. Available at http://www.hpc-uk.org

Health and Care Professions Council (2005) Standards for Continuing Professional Development [Online] HCPC. Available at http://www.hpc-uk.org

Leonard, M, Graham, S and Bonacum, D The human factor: the critical importance of effective teamwork and communication in providing safe care. *Quality & Safety in Health Care* 2014; 13 (1) 85–90.

Little, P, et al. Observational study of effect of patient centredness and positive approach on outcomes of general practice consultations. *British Medical Journal* 2001; 323(7381); 908–11.

McCormack, B and McCance, T (2010) *Person-Centred Nursing: Theory and Practice. Ed. Chichester: Wiley-Blackwell.*

NHS Institute of Innovation and Improvement, Plan Do Study Act toolkit [Online] Available at www.institute.nhs.uk/quality_and_service_improvement_tools/quality_and_service_improvement_tools/plan_do_study_act.html [Accessed October, 2012].

Nursing and Midwifery Council (2010) The code: Standards of conduct, performance and ethics for nurses and midwives. Nursing and Midwifery Council. [Online] Available at www.standards.nmc-uk.org/

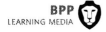

Nursing and Midwifery Council (2004) *Midwives Rules and Standards. London:* NMC Publications.

Royal College Of Obstetrics and Gynaecology (2007) *Management of genital herpes in pregnancy. Guideline No 30.* RCOG Press.

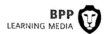

Chapter 8

Leadership learning at post-qualifying stage in the ward

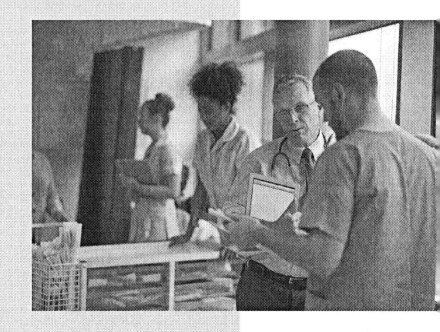

Chapter 8

Leadership learning at post-qualifying stage in the ward

Chapter overview

This chapter provides:

- A description of post-qualifying learning and how it relates to the five domains of the CLCF.

- Ward based culture and leadership.

- Five case studies describing leadership in practice.

Introduction

At the practitioner and experienced practitioner stage of the CLCF clinicians will most likely be working. The context of their clinical practice will depend on their discipline or specialty. It may be in the NHS or the private sector. Although all clinicians work within a system, many will be working independently or possibly remotely from colleagues. The CLCF is designed to be applicable where you are working. In the next chapters we explore leadership at a post qualifying stage.

Ward based leadership

Acute environments such as wards and cardiac and intensive care units have permanent nursing staff. However many other professions such as doctors and other allied professionals are transient making continuity of care a significant challenge for all involved. A solution to this issue has come in the form of integrated care pathways (ICP). Interest has grown in ICPs due to healthcare imperatives such as more efficient use of resources, improvement in quality of care and expanding best practice, the desire for automation of health records and the quest for better ways to engage patients and their families (Zander, 2002).

Organisational culture can also impact on the experience and outcomes for patients. Organisational culture in a hospital is not a single entity rather it is composed of many disparate professional

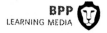

cultures such as medicine, nursing, allied health and management and within these further subcultures such as surgery, pharmacy and finance (Carroll & Quijada, 2004). It is also important to recognise the international cultures that exist within hospitals. A culture change takes a long time and it is important to bring people together with a common purpose that appeals to ethical values & beliefs and there is an emerging call for authentic leaders (Northouse, 2010).

Within the acute setting many teams are necessitated to provide holistic care to patients, their families and/or carers. Health professionals need to respect each other and work together to maintain safe, high quality care for patients.

Whilst hospitals provide a rich environment for all health professionals to develop their leadership and management skills making use of these opportunities is a challenge when time can be limited and the demand of workloads can be exhausting.

Demonstrating Personal Qualities

One of the principal personal qualities of a leader is self-awareness. Being aware of one's own beliefs, attitudes and assumptions and learning from experience. As individuals move from the early years post registration, or qualifying to the more experienced stage of their career they will become more aware of themselves, of their own values, principles and assumptions, learning from their experiences. These will change and evolve as their career progresses and as they hold more complex roles and have greater responsibility. Developing a culture of feedback and suggestions from all those involved regarding improvements in care can be an influential way of galvanising teams.

Working with Others

As indicated the culture of an organisation can impact significantly on patient care and outcomes. Historically, hierarchies within an organisation have impacted on team work. Providing safe care is reliant on effective communication and teamwork and all too frequently patient harm is the result of poor communication (Leonard *et al*; 2004). With the adoption of distributed leadership a more shared approach to leadership is encouraged, respecting the views and contributions of all staff. No one health care profession can provide for all the needs of a patient, providing holistic care for individual patients requires

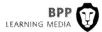

integrated, seamless services and this can only be accomplished through effective team work. Health care has seen an erosion of professional boundaries in recent years with the introduction of the European Working Time Directive the traditional roles of health care professionals have dissipated with nursing and other allied professionals taking on roles formerly associated with doctors.

The service users have a right to expect healthcare practitioners to work effectively within multi-professional teams and also equally effectively across and between agencies. The patients' benefit from practitioners maintaining and strengthening these relationships with the aim of providing a seamless service. Effective working with others helps to achieve a good clinical outcome in a timely and accurate way. For example patient discharge is a key process that demands established networks that value and respect other groups or agencies decisions. In this situation it is essential that the healthcare professional translates these ideologies into practice for the benefit of the service user and their families and carers.

Managing Services

At this stage of their career all clinicians need to be involved in managing services. This does not necessarily mean in a positional sense or managerial role, though increasingly in the modern NHS staff employed at Bands 6 and 7 are required to manage some aspect of the service.

Within the climate of financial pressures all professions need to manage resources effectively and efficiently developing knowledge and skills in this area will support the wider organisation to be more successful. By virtue of their unique role in the allocation and utilisation of resources, such as diagnostic tests, expensive therapies, procedures and operations, and use of consumables including costly drugs all clinicians need to be able to be competent at managing services and resources. For example, it should be possible to reduce expensive hospital admissions by getting patients more involved in managing their own conditions, where possible and treating more patients closer to home.

As well as managing resources people management is central to this area of responsibility ensuring the right person doing the right thing in the right place at the right time is central to a streamlined service, reducing duplication of effort and removing unnecessary steps in the patient pathway serves to enhance patient experience and outcomes.

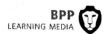

Improving Services

Healthcare practitioners are required to maintain and where possible enhance the quality and productivity of the service. Adopting a culture of continuous improvement across services can help to maintain impetus for improving services. Familiarity with service improvement techniques such as six sigma or lean methodologies can support the development of high quality care. This transformation and culture shift can be stifled by traditions and historical practices. Professionals need to adopt attitudes and behaviours that encourage a culture of continuous improvement.

The NHS Quality Innovation Prevention and Productivity (QIPP) initiative is an approach to improving services that supports the practitioner to maintain quality while innovating the service and increasing productivity. Frontline clinical leaders will play a key role in promoting QIPP as they have first-hand experience and knowledge of the areas where QIPP will make a difference (Department of Health, 2011). Specific activities such as clinical audit and research will be vital to the successful outcome of the QIPP and improving all services.

Setting Direction

As valued and well established members of staff or as partners, or a team member, all clinicians are able to develop further their leadership abilities by actively contributing to the running of the organisation and to the way care is provided generally. Wider strategic direction of an organisation is usually set by policy and executive board members, however operating within wards and departments offers professionals the opportunity to identify areas for change, applying relevant knowledge and evidence and participating in and contributing to operational decision making.

Clinical leadership comes from the need to understand how their speciality and focus of care contributes to the wider healthcare system. Their familiarity with their specific focus of care enables them to work outside their immediate setting and to look further at ways to improve the experience of healthcare for patients and colleagues.

The following five case studies illustrate the practitioner and experienced practitioner examples and how leadership is applicable to the context of their clinical practice. At this level of experience

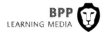

many CLCF competences have become embedded and are often used implicitly. Nearly all of the CLCF domains are used at some point and it is important the reader cross references to the CLCF to see how the different competences mentioned in the text cohere to provide examples of leadership.

Continuing personal and professional development

Most clinicians undertake continuing professional development and workplace learning (Department of Health, 2012) and consider it a core part of the commitment as a professional and as part of their revalidation. All these areas now include significant aspects of leadership development based on the CLCF.

Regulatory bodies require all registered practitioners to demonstrate their continued competence through regular continuing professional development (Long and Spurgeon, 2012). The Health and Care Professions Council (HCPC) defines Continuing Professional Development (CPD) as:

'A range of learning activities through which health professionals maintain and develop throughout their career to ensure that they retain their capacity to practice safely, effectively and legally within their evolving scope of practice.' (HCPC, 2009)

The HCPC recently released a position statement concerning leadership with particular reference to the CLCF:

'We consider that the CLCF is important in helping clinicians to develop a shared understanding of what leadership is and in aiming to develop leadership behaviours at all levels of seniority' (HCPC, 2012)

As part of their on-going competence maintenance and enhanced skill development the qualified clinician should reflect on the five core domains of the CLCF and identify where and when in their daily clinical practice they use the behaviours identified in the framework. This approach ensures that a practitioner takes their own responsibility for ensuring they can evidence the characteristics identified by these elements within the core domains. This approach will also guarantee that staff will develop shared leadership skills and understand they have a shared leadership responsibility for the success of the organisation and the services it provides (HCPC, 2012).

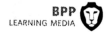

The way that the CLCF applies to an individual will depend on the service they deliver and the role they have in an organisation.

Case Study 1 Challenging for improvement

Part of the role of a clinical engineering practitioner was to look after specialised laser equipment in one of the hospital's day theatres, providing day to day operational support and maintenance. On one of his regular visits junior theatre staff asked him if he knew anything about changes to the facility, as they had heard rumours that the theatre was going to be used for something else. He asked each of his clinical colleagues in the child dermatology and plastics treatment sessions but they had heard nothing.

The clinical engineer realised that alterations to the operating theatre could affect the safety adaptations that were needed for laser use, such as blinds to shield windows and warning lights to show the laser was operational. He approached the theatre manager to ask what was happening and found out there were plans to decommission the existing theatre and move its activity to one dedicated to plastics, as part of a larger reconfiguration project. No-one had told the existing users and the service manager was not aware a patient laser was being used. Although this was not the engineer's area of responsibility, he decided he would take action to prevent patient treatment being disrupted (Element 1(iv) Acting with integrity).

After further enquiries with the clinical users and theatre managers, the engineer clarified (Element 5(i) Evaluating impact) that no alternative arrangements had been made for patient laser treatments, no-one had realised the legal need for safety precautions and there was no provision for moving the laser equipment between the two theatres or storing it safely. Moreover the change was due to happen in less than a month to meet the overall building timetable.

The engineer talked to a number of staff to identify who was responsible for managing the different laser procedures and facilities. He talked to three different service managers and their staff about how their services worked now and how that could change (Element 2(i) Developing networks). He quickly investigated various technical possibilities with the Works department and then submitted a proposal to all the parties involved suggesting what could be done to enable treatment to continue (Element 5(ii) Applying knowledge and evidence). There was no progress until he sent a follow up email highlighting the fact that patient appointments would have to be cancelled if nothing was done. This led to a flurry of emails and although the project to decommission the theatre had just started, he managed to negotiate a week's delay with the internal project manager and external contractor (Element 4(iv) Innovation and facilitating transformation). He arranged for the partly stripped out room to be made safe for clinical procedures and to be deep cleaned over a weekend,

---

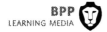

then put the equipment back and checked everything was safe and working correctly first thing on the Monday morning so that no patient treatments had to be cancelled that week (Element 4(i) Ensuring patient safety). He then arranged for the Works department to install warning lights and power supplies into the alternative plastics theatre the next Saturday and for it to be deep cleaned on the Sunday, and moved the equipment in early Monday morning to get it ready for patients later that day.

Although this had dealt with the immediate crisis and prevented patient treatments being affected, he was concerned about the longer term issue of children's work being carried out in an adult theatre (Element 4(ii) Critically evaluating). However, when he raised the issue the theatre matron and other managers told him they had previously tried to get a theatre in the children's hospital converted for laser usage but had been told it would take around two years for it to be done. He decided to try to change this situation (Element 1(iv) Acting with integrity) and researched whether any special requirements were needed and what was already in place. He found that two recently installed modular theatres dedicated to child services already had laser lights and blinds installed as standard. He asked the children's theatre manager to review the workload and found it was possible for them to fit the appropriate dermatology work into the theatre lists. He arranged with the works department to install the necessary power supplies in both theatres the following weekend, to allow for future flexibility (Element 3(ii) Managing resources), set up the deep cleaning and arranged to come in early on the Monday to put the equipment in place. Then a colleague pointed out that procedures could not go ahead without suitable nursing support in place, so he called a meeting with the dermatology nursing staff and managers to reach an understanding of what the problems were (Element 2(iv) Working within teams). This led to a suitable recovery space being set up in the children's hospital (Element 4(iii) Encouraging improvement). He also set up tours of the new theatre so that the dermatology staff would be introduced to the children's theatre staff and facilities they would be working with, and demonstrated the equipment to the theatre nurses (Element 2(i) Developing networks).

He presented the lessons he had learnt to his colleagues (Element 1(iii) Continuing personal development) and asked for feedback from those he had worked with (Element 1(i) Developing self-awareness). In summary, he found it was necessary to continue to be involved at every stage and to contact people directly rather than relying on emails. He had also learnt it was important to be clear and direct in conversation (Element 1(iv) Acting with integrity) and to try to understand what individuals' constraints were. In the process of achieving the end goal of ensuring uninterrupted patient treatment he worked with over 20 internal staff and an outside contractor and improved the use of hospital resources and the quality of patient services.

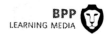

Case Study 2 Providing support to individual colleagues whilst managing organisational performance

The following case is a challenging, multifaceted scenario which highlights many issues relating to mental distress in a colleague. The case illustrates how a practitioner or experienced practitioner can use the CLCF to support a colleague, learn from the experience to understand if other colleagues are experiencing similar problems and spread the learning to the wider organisation.

Derek is a clinical psychologist working in a mental health service at a NHS trust. A colleague Ellen is a qualified nurse and works part-time at the same NHS hospital in a High Dependency/ Intensive Care unit. Ellen is 34 years old and is a married woman with two adolescent children. Her husband, James, who is fifteen years older than Ellen, is a consultant surgeon at a local NHS hospital. Outwardly to colleagues, friends and family they are respected, well-liked and happy but Derek is aware from conversations with Ellen that in private James can be very demanding and difficult with occasional bouts of anger.

Ellen was involved in a road traffic accident some six months previously whilst travelling back from a late shift. At the time she was driving her husband's new car as her own car was under repair. Ellen's health has deteriorated in the months following the accident and Derek is aware that she has not been eating properly and has lost a significant amount of weight. She is experiencing episodes of poor sleep and frequent nightmares. She is often visibly distressed and she has been leaving work early to avoid driving through the intersection where the accident took place because it makes her feel panicky. Consequently she now goes home a different way from work. However this adds a further 20 minutes onto her journey so Ellen is leaving her Intensive Care Unit early. Although her colleagues were initially supportive of Ellen post-accident her leaving early means that Ellen does not participate in handovers between staff. This is now causing Ellen problems at work with disharmony with her colleagues. One of Ellen's colleagues at work is threatening to inform their manager that Ellen is leaving the unit early.

Using the domains and elements and behaviours of the CLCF we can understand how Derek exercised leadership to address this case.

As a lead clinician in the Trust Derek has a role in managing services (CLCF Domain 3). Although not directly involved Derek decides to speak to Ellen about her situation to support her and see if he is able to help in some way (Element 3(iii) Managing People). Recognising this may be a difficult conversation out of respect for Ellen, Derek arranges to meet her in his office, where he can be sure that their discussions will be confidential and she will feel comfortable (CLCF Domain 1 Demonstrating Personal Qualities).

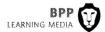

Apparently Ellen was subsequently late home from work the night of the accident and when Ellen tried to explain the reason for her being late, seeing the damage to the car James was verbally abusive to Ellen referring to her as a 'stupid, stupid woman who can't do anything right' before slapping her hard around the face. Although Ellen has always been faithful in her marriage, James later explained his behaviour down to he'd been thinking she was late because she was having an affair with another man.

At the time of this incident both children witnessed their mum being shouted at and being assaulted by their father and when Ellen recounted how distressed the children where that night, she became massively distressed.

During the discussion Ellen eventually discloses many years of domestic violence perpetrated by James. Ellen also discloses that she has contemplated taking her own life and feels that this is the only option open to her at times. She is extremely anxious now at driving and has frequent headaches and panic attacks.

Recognising that this is a very complex situation which cannot easily be resolved Derek takes care not to show his own emotions about the situation and works with Ellen to help her feel supported and understand how she can work through her issues (Element 1(ii) Managing themselves and Element 3(iii) Managing People). Concerned that Ellen may self-harm Derek immediately arranges for her to see another colleague for a proper mental health assessment. He also makes Ellen aware of the Trust Employee Assistance Programme (EAP) which is available for all staff and offers a free, confidential and independent counselling service. (CLCF 1 Demonstrating Personal Qualities and CLCF 3(i) Managing people).

While acting to support Ellen, Derek is also aware of the broader consequences of the case to the delivery of safe care for patients and that there is a potential patient safety issue. With Ellen's consent, he contacts her manager to let him know that Ellen is experiencing difficulties and together they organise for Ellen to do her hand-over earlier until she is sufficiently well again to drive home via the shorter route (Domain 2 Working With Others and Element 4(i) Ensuring patient safety).

On a personal level, Derek showed sensitivity for colleagues with differing views and when he was leading the discussions always listened and ensured discussions were open, accepting and positive, and that all ideas were welcome. When a doctor voiced an opinion that there was no benefit in including patients in the survey Derek challenged this view as being contrary to the Trust's aim of working in partnership with people who use services, and emphasised his own experience and viewpoint that their voice was invaluable in understanding if the service was meeting their needs (Element 1(iv) Acting with integrity). He was also able to support his viewpoint by using data from

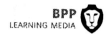

the national survey of junior staff that showed evidence of junior medical staff being bullyied and harassed by senior doctors at some NHS trusts (Element 3(iv) Managing Performance).

The survey went ahead and indicated 30% of respondents had experienced or were aware that staff are experiencing forms of impairment such as distress. The Trust senior management appointed Derek as the lead in reviewing policy and procedures for supporting impaired staff, and to work with stakeholders on a campaign to raise awareness of impaired practitioners and how colleagues can support each other and high quality care (Element 3(iv) Managing performance).

Case Study 3 Leadership for improved patient safety

While working within her role as Clinical Operations Manager/Matron in a Tertiary Cardiac Centre, Angela worked on a service improvement project for patients undergoing coronary intervention within the day case department in a tertiary centre hospital trust. During the project she referred to the (CLCF) to help inform her actions and decisions. The following case study illustrates how clinical leadership can be demonstrated with reference to CLCF elements. The case study demonstrates leadership particularly in the Domains: 2 Working with others, 4 Improving Services and 5 Setting Direction.

Angela identified the context for change (Element 5(i) Identifying the contexts for change) as she was aware that in her hospital on average 10-12 cardiac patients presented for day case coronary intervention procedures. Approximately half of them were being admitted to the inpatient area but at least four to five of these patients were discharged home the same day and Angela sought to improve the experience of these patients. Angela looked at the current knowledge and evidence (Element 5(ii) Applying knowledge and evidence) and was aware there was no national information regarding day case procedures for patient undergoing coronary intervention however she accessed European benchmark data which included information about Amsterdam's radial lounge model, this helped inform the decision making process (Element 5(iii) Making decisions).

Coronary angiography is a day case procedure but Percutaneous Coronary Intervention (PCI) has historically involved admission to hospital and an overnight stay after the procedure. It has been shown that same day discharge after PCI can be performed safely in selected patients. With the introduction of a radial lounge, patients will be admitted to and subsequently discharged on the same day from a dedicated area – containing only chairs – thereby avoiding the need to access a hospital bed at any time.

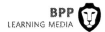

While in the lounge, patients will have access to telephones, internet points and televisions allowing them to continue with many aspects of their day-to-day lives. The aim of the radial lounge is to accommodate patients in an attractive environment before and after their procedure in a way that minimises the feeling of 'hospitalisation' that accompanies most encounters with health services.

Angela recognised that to encourage improvement (Element 4(iii)) and facilitate change (Element 4(iv)) she would need to engage staff, she encouraged contribution from others (Element 2(iii)) and worked with her team (Element 2(iii)) to analyse the current situation. The team used a process mapping tool and walked the patient journey listening to the patient voice. As a result Angela and her team critically evaluated (Element 4(ii)) the current service and identified four steps in the process which could be improved and would impact on patient experience and bed utilisation.

To effectively manage the implementation of the radial lounge Angela used the PDSA cycle, this enabled Angela to plan effectively for the change (Element 3(i)) by communicating with staff and patients, introducing new policies and procedures, ensuring patient safety by developing appropriate selection criteria for the radial lounge (Element 4(i)), evaluating the change (Element 5(iv)) and reporting findings of the project to the hospital's resuscitation committee.

Key learning points from the case study are appreciating change cannot be made by an individual and for change to be successful you need to work within teams (Element 2(iv)). Ensuring patient safety (Element 4(i)) at times of change is also critical this is enhanced through clear communication and effective planning (Element 3(i)).

Case Study 4 Learning and improving by listening to patients and staff

As a supervisor of midwives Julie has a responsibility to ensure high quality care for women by ensuring midwives are competent to practice. Supervision is a statutory role and all practicing midwives must have a named supervisor of midwives whom they meet at least annually and whenever necessary in between.

Whilst working within this role Julie along with the other midwife supervisors identified a service improvement need. Julie and her colleagues referred to the CLCF framework to aid their actions and decisions. The case study below highlights leadership behaviours particularly in Domains 2 Working with others, 4 Improving services and 5. Setting direction.

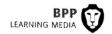

One of the challenges faced by Julie in her role as a Midwife Supervisor is the engagement of users in order to illicit feedback on their services. In order to improve the experience of users and encourage improvement (Element 4(iii)) Julie and her colleagues started to 'walk the floor' on a regular basis, getting feedback from women on their service and any issues.

As a consequence of this feedback together with additional feedback from the annual Local Supervisory Authority audit (LSA), Julie and the team commenced a pilot project allowing partners to stay overnight with their partner once the baby is born.

The proposal represented a significant change in practice for the midwives. Julie recognised the change would need support from the midwives themselves for it to be successful, and in order to encourage contribution (Element 2(iii)) from others and working within the wider team (Element 2(iv)) a survey of women and midwives' views was undertaken to identify issues and address any concerns that arose. The survey helped to identify the context for change (Element 5(i)) and making decisions (Element 5(iii)) regarding changes to policies and procedures.

The survey garnered two diverse views. The expectant women were very positive and thought it was a very good idea; the midwives were more reluctant, fearing issues with partners at night, partners requiring a place to sleep and expecting food and beverages.

Julie and her colleagues addressed the issues raised by the midwives individually building relationships (2(ii)) and encouraging improvement (4(iii)). The result was a contract between partners and the labour ward. Partners would sign to agree that they will only have a chair by the bed and must not sleep on other beds, beverages are available but no food and that any aggressive behaviour will not be tolerated.

The project is currently in the pilot phase and its impact will be evaluated (Element 5(iv)) to ensure the change has had a positive impact on all concerned and any issues raised have been mitigated. Julie and the team of supervisors have continued to 'walk the floor' and have received very positive feedback from the women and partners. The midwives have also reported mostly positive feedback, saying that the partners who stay overnight are often very helpful, assisting their partners and reducing the women's anxiety. Engaging the midwives from an early stage enabled the facilitation of change (Element 4(iv)). Garnering the views of their service users and using this to influence decision making (Element 5(iii)) and service improvement (Element 4(iv)) has made a real difference to the experiences of women in the labour ward.

Key learning points from this experience include the need to engage and listen to feedback from service users and how this can be instrumental in affecting change. Encouraging contribution (2(iii)) from staff and working within teams (2(iv)) can facilitate sustainable service improvements that are owned by staff.

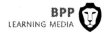

Case Study 5 Transforming a service through technical and leadership skills

Keith, a qualified Pharmacist, recently took up a position managing a busy Pharmacy in a City centre. He leads a team consisting of another pharmacist, two pharmacy technicians and three healthcare assistants. Shortly after starting his new position, he noticed he was frequently getting requests for travel health advice by patients travelling overseas. Feedback from patients suggested the provision of travel health services locally was patchy. It was clear that many members of the community were not receiving the best healthcare prior to travelling overseas.

Keith is a keen traveller himself and he understands the risks and implications of travelling without receiving the right vaccinations. This was unacceptable in opinion and he set out to understand what he could do to address this (Element 5(i) Identifying the contexts for change).

Keith referred to the CLCF to help inform his actions and decisions. The following case study illustrates how clinical leadership can be demonstrated by a practitioner with reference to CLCF elements. The case study demonstrates that Keith's work shows leadership particularly in the Domains: 2 Working with others, 3 Managing Services, 4 Improving Services.

Keith contacted local healthcare practitioners and commissioners to discuss travel health provisions. His findings confirmed there are very few local NHS practices offering the range of vaccinations required by travellers. Where there was provision, available appointment slots were limited. He wanted to understand why this was the case. He followed up discussions with a number of GPs and nurses who provided this service; it was clear travel health was seen as a low priority and consequently clinical updates and best practices were not always adopted. Furthermore he held meetings with pharmaceutical industry contacts to understand the private healthcare market (Element 2(i) Developing networks). It was clear there was an opportunity to establish a private In-Pharmacy Travel Clinic.

Keith researched into the legal framework for establishing a travel health service. Working in partnership with an Independent Medical Agency (IMA), he set about creating a comprehensive In-Pharmacy Travel Clinic adopting a Patient Group Directive (PGD) model (Element 4(iii) Encouraging improvement). He started by developing the PGDs and clinical governance for the service. The IMA and Keith consulted regulatory bodies and professional bodies prior to signing off the final version of the service specification (Element 3(i) Planning).

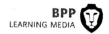

Having established the legal framework and clinical governance for the service, Keith spent a period of time developing an implementation plan, with clear timelines and markers in place in order to launch date. He sought feedback from his team and was able to make amends accordingly.

Having previously received training on managing anaphylaxis and vaccination technique (intramuscular), Keith realised he still needed training on other routes of administration. He arranged a one to one vaccination technique training session with his local practice nurse (Element 1(iii) Continuing professional development).

Keith identified the lack of Yellow Fever centres locally so he attended NAthNac training and accredited his pharmacy as a Yellow Fever centre. He also attended a two day training workshop which enabled him to develop a specialism in Travel Health and understand where to find further resources, subscribing to current Travel Health websites such as Travax.

Keith understood the importance of conducting an in-depth quality travel risk assessment with his patients prior to administering the vaccinations. He reviewed the various different risk assessment forms and, in partnership with the IMA, developed a bespoke version for use in his practice. To ensure his patients received the best care in his pharmacy, he made adjustments to his consulting room enabling him to manage any potential adverse effects anaphylaxis (Element 4(i) Ensuring patient safety).

Keith believed it was important to engage with the local healthcare community and ensure his service is joined-up linking in with current NHS providers. He made appointments to visit all GP practices locally to discuss the service (Element 4(iv) Innovation and facilitating transformation). As part of his visit, Keith established pathways for referrals (Element 2(i) Developing networks). He created a pathway document, which was refined following feedback from GP and nurse colleagues. He sent out the final version to all practices.

Keith was slightly surprised however to learn of concerns from a small number of nurses based on perceived 'competition' and 'private sector health services'. He listened to their concerns, and explained in detail, the complementary nature of the service which provided patients choice and improved access. Additionally as he had developed a specialism, he offered the GP and nurse colleagues the option of being able to contact him at any time, should they wish to discuss or refer complex cases. This offer was warmly received by all, and concerns were addressed (Element 2(ii) Building and maintaining networks). He received up to 8 phone calls per week from his colleagues.

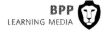

> Shortly after launch, Keith realised there was a higher demand for the service than he had anticipated. He realised that the service often involved the pharmacist being away from the dispensary for up to 30 minutes per appointment, and this was consequently affecting the delivery of core pharmaceutical services. He identified the need to amend his team's skill mix and update his training and succession plans accordingly. A technician was enrolled onto an accuracy checking technician course, and a plan was in place for the new skill mix to be in place within 8 weeks (Element 3(ii) Managing resources), (Element 3(iii) Managing people), (3(iv) Managing performance).
>
> Keith decided this was an excellent opportunity to gather quality patient feedback in order to help improve his current service as well as to generate evidence to inform future commissioners of the viability of commissioning vaccination services in his pharmacy. He created a patient feedback form which when completed, could be inputted into a database.
>
> Within a period of weeks, Keith was able to build up sufficient data in order for him to analyse and make changes accordingly. Examples included an amended process for booking appointments, and stocking a wider range of travel health products (mosquito nets). (Element 5(iv) Evaluating impact). Armed with the quality data, he will be discussing the service with future commissioners. Widely accepted as a travel health specialist, Keith now delivers talks on the subject to local practices, universities and businesses.

Chapter summary

In this chapter we learned:

- Within the acute setting many teams are necessitated to provide holistic care to patients, their families and/or carers.

- Hospital wards provide a rich and diverse range of opportunities for clinicians to develop their leadership skills and practice.

- Team working and shared leadership is a challenge when time is limited and the demand of workloads exhausting.

- Health professionals need to respect each other and work together to maintain safe, high quality care for patients.

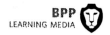

Three things to try

1. Participate in peer learning and explore team and leadership styles and preferences.

2. Start a conversation about developing care pathways.

3. Take part in departmental discussions about resource allocation and service improvement.

Chapter references

Carroll, J, S, and Quijada, M, A. Redirecting traditional professional values to support safety: changing organisational culture in health care. *Quality and Safety Health Care 2004; 13 (16).*

Department of Health (2011). The Operating Framework for the NHS in England 2012/13. Department of Health.

Department of Health (2012). Liberating the NHS: Developing the Healthcare Workforce from Design to Delivery *Gateway Reference* 16977.

Health Care Professions Council (2012) HCPC Position Statement on NHS Clinical Leadership Competency Framework. HCPC. [Online] Available at HYPERLINK "http://www.hpc-uk.org/ assets/documents/10003C4404-positionstatementonleadership. pdf"www.hpc-uk.org/assets/documents/10003C4404-positionstatementonleadership.pdf

Leonard, M, Graham, S and Bonacum, D. The human factor: the critical importance of effective teamwork and communication in providing safe care. *BMJ Quality and Safety 2004; 13(Suppl. 1) 85–90.*

Long P, W, Spurgeon, P, C. Embedding leadership into professional, regulatory and educational standards. *International Journal of Clinical Leadership 2012; 17, (4).*

Northouse, P G (2010) Leadership: Theory and practice, *eds.,* London: SAGE

Zander, K. Integrated Care Pathways: eleven international trends, *Journal of Integrated Care Pathways 2002; 6, 101–107.*

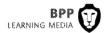

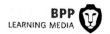

Chapter 9

Leadership in the community/ primary care

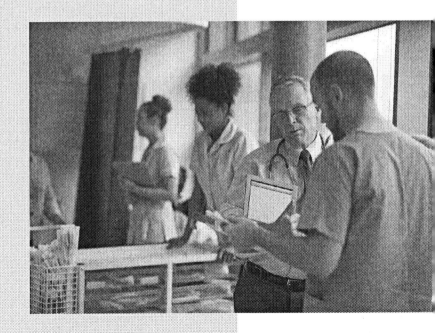

Leadership in the community/primary care

Chapter overview

This chapter provides:

- Leadership in the community and primary care setting and how it relates to the 5 domains of the CLCF.

- Four case studies describing leadership in practice.

Introduction

With the transformation of services in the acute setting comes the need to change services in primary care. The high cost of acute care and the reduction of acute beds means patients need to be cared for in their own home and the health care system is being restructured to be more primary care focused with greater emphasis on prevention, self-care and integrated primary and community care (Goodwin *et al*; 2011). Providing services that keep people out of hospital is challenging particularly with an ever aging population living with multiple co morbidities. Primary care is facing one of its greatest challenges with devolvement of budgets to Clinical Commissioning Groups affording primary care clinicians a greater input in to how funding is spent, whilst providing and developing services for patients is exigent and will require significant leadership capability.

Demonstrating Personal Qualities

As with all other areas of healthcare, clinicians need to manage self and demonstrate a high degree of self-awareness. In primary care where often there is little back up it can be argued that delivering care to patients is inherently riskier and therefore potentially invokes additional stress. Clinical staff work mainly on their own experiencing varying degrees of access to support mechanisms with limited opportunity to discuss issues or problems that occur during the working day. Managing self in this environment becomes ever more crucial.

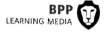

Working with Others

Maintaining people in their own homes can often involve a wide range of professionals with their own respective caseloads. Delivering safe and effective care in the community requires these professional groups to work together transcending professional and organisational boundaries, building networks that are patient-centred. It is easy for managerial hierarchies to become and appear disengaged from frontline care and the problems that arise. It is the responsibility of everyone engaged in community care to nurture and sustain an effective network of services from cradle to grave.

Managing Services

Managing successful services in the community requires excellent planning skills and this is imperative with an ever increasing complex case load. Effective planning ensures good use of resources including equipment and people, timely intervention and reduces delayed or duplication of care. Without co-ordination and planning of primary and community care services the quality and cost effectiveness of care can diminish (Kodner & Spreeuwenberg, 2002).

Improving Services

Significant transformational changes to the health care system are creating opportunities to improve the way services are delivered. New care pathways are paving the way for one stop solutions, easier access and streamlined services. Nursing and allied professionals have been at the forefront of these developments, adopting change methodologies and implementing evidenced based or good practice initiatives. As the system is dynamic a culture of continuous improvement needs to pervade the service.

Setting Direction

Applying knowledge and evidence to primary and community care services is central to setting direction. It is no longer acceptable to do something because it's the way it has always been done. Applying the evidence base entails data and information gathering, analysis, using data to challenge current practice and inspiring others to apply knowledge and evidence to attain best practice.

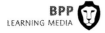

Evidence-based medicine in the form of national and local guidelines exist for most clinical conditions and it is important clinicians continue to question the evidence and add to the knowledge base in order to further improve practice.

Case Study 1 Managing your personal development within a work context

Sue is the Clinical Pharmacy Manager at a 850 bed Acute Hospital Trust where she manages a team of 114 staff. Sue is directly accountable to the Director of Pharmacy and acts as his deputy in his absence. She has a demanding and complex role which requires her to demonstrate high level leadership behaviours. Whilst concentrating on her day to day role in a large and challenging organisation, she is also mindful of her own career development and what skills and abilities she needs to develop to become a Director of Pharmacy in the future. She has used the Leadership Competency Framework for Pharmacy Professionals, which has the same domains and elements as the CLCF, to structure her development and to guide her (Royal Pharmaceutical Society, 2011).

She has used the competency framework to structure her development over the past year alongside becoming a member of an Action Learning Set group with peers. She has used frameworks before but found that the domains included in this particular framework aligned more closely to her current personal development needs. In choosing to use the framework, she has been able to be specific about which leadership behaviours she wished to develop. This case study illustrates her development across a number of domains in the framework and some of the tools and techniques she used to support her development and includes examples from her practice.

The examples reference the domains in the framework:

Element 1(i) Developing Self Awareness

Sue had been increasingly aware that her very busy role had increasingly impacted on her time and her ability to be consistent in her approach to all her staff. She had not thought about the way her behaviour could influence others in any detail.

She used one of the tools recommended in the framework to identify methods to address this. She undertook a 360° review using an accredited tool. This provided some insightful and useful feedback. Some of this she felt she could predict and some feedback she was not expecting. She was aware that she needed to be open and accepting of this feedback and then be prepared to look for ways to change. She had not had this type of feedback in 20 years of experience of team working.

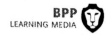

Element 1(iii) Continuing Professional Development

Sue was one of the most senior members of her department but was finding it difficult to get feedback on her performance and development from anywhere outside the normal appraisal process. She used the examples in the framework to secure the support from a mentor. She chose a senior member of the hospital management team. They met monthly for six months. Sue found this a very useful exercise. Her mentor was able to help her review examples in the framework and how she could apply those to her practice.

Element 2(iii) Encouraging Contribution

Sue has a strong senior management team who have recently been working on introducing a new working hours policy. The policy has required members of the team to roll out a 24/7 working pattern in their sub teams. Many of the senior team felt very strongly about this and as such were making the implementation meetings very challenging. Sue reviewed the framework and thought about what behaviours she could influence to provide a better outcome. She tried a new technique and met briefly with each individual to hear their concerns. She then produced a draft document which she circulated before the meeting. Subsequently the meeting ran well and major arguments were avoided as most of the major issues had been reviewed and discussed in advance. The meeting gained consensus and the policy was introduced with minimal controversy. Sue felt that the more strategic way of managing conflicts of interest had allowed differences of opinion to be considered and had met her personal objective of introducing this complex policy.

Element 4(i) Ensuring Patient Safety

Sue has been the lead in redesigning and implementing a new Trust medication chart. This is a complex process which involves implementation of national guidelines and involves multiple teams and departments from the organisation. Sue undertook training from the Safer Patients Initiative and then used small cycles of change to implement the new chart. She tested them on one ward with one group of patients and then rolled this out. She was keen to try this new technique and felt that the framework helped her to use systematic ways to assess the risk and review the impact of changes.

Summary

Sue used a series of Action Learning Sets with peers to help her focus on which aspects of the Leadership Framework for pharmacy professionals she was developing. With a senior role in a complex organisation, Sue was able to develop varied and complementary leadership abilities. She also had time over the course of a year to appreciate how many of the domains are linked and influence the others and how these few examples are just the starting point for many more.

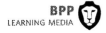

Learning context for others – How could this case help you?

Have you thought about how your behaviours influence others in your team? Perhaps 360° feedback could help you to obtain feedback on your own leadership style? Remember to ensure you are able to get an experienced facilitator to help you to interpret it.

Have you ever thought about having a mentor? Could someone outside your department fulfil this role? Consider the additional value that a non-pharmacist could bring to your development.

Do you struggle to bring people with you on a big project? Do you have a team to manage full of big personalities and strong views? Consider implementing strategies that allow their views to be considered but maintain a focus on your patient facing objectives.

Have you had to implement part of the patient safety agenda across other multiple departments and teams that you do not directly manage? Consider a more strategic approach to implementing change. Look out for techniques and tools from organisations such as the Institute for Healthcare Improvement (IHI) or the new NHS Improving Quality body, which is part of NHS England.

Case Study 2 Working across boundaries to address patient concerns

The National Service Framework for Older Adults had advocated a single assessment process and the sharing of information across agencies in order to integrate care and the services provided in the local area, and to create a more efficient and meaningful process for patients and carers. Locally, a survey of the views of patients and carers had clearly identified how annoyed they got when they were asked the same questions by different professions who didn't seem to know what their colleagues were doing, know of details previous shared with others, or adequately communicate safety issues with each other.

Pat was Head Occupational Therapist for a team of occupational therapists working in the field of care of the elderly mentally ill across a large geographical area, they supported people in the community with both functional mental illnesses, such as depression and anxiety, and also people suffering from dementia to live as independent a life as possible, they also supported carers.

The team worked very closely with colleagues from many different spheres and local organisations: psychologists, specialist nursing colleagues (in-patient and community teams), social workers, medical staff, general practitioners, nursing and therapy colleagues in the general hospital, the voluntary sector and charities.

 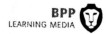

Pat and the team actively took part in changing the way the needs of older adults in the local area were assessed, recorded and shared with colleagues. In doing so, Pat demonstrated a positive and constructive contribution to the leadership of the whole service and the shared goals of achieving a better provision of care for everyone, patients and carers. (Element 2(ii) Building and maintaining relationships).

Using the domains, elements and behaviours of the CLCF, it is possible to look more closely at how that contribution was made.

Pat was able to describe the urgency and need to improve the local services, this included ensuring patient/service user and carer safety, especially in the residential setting; supporting the critical evaluation of existing practice and how the various professions and services interacted and communicated; creating a culture and climate that encouraged change and improvement; and in working with senior colleagues to embed and role model the required changes in practice (Element 4(ii) Critically evaluating, 5(i) Identifying the contexts for change and 5(ii) Applying knowledge and evidence).

The change process included large scale events to which all parties were invited to contribute in an active way; to take a blank sheet and look at the process from the patient/service user viewpoint. Pat was able to encourage and role model both the creativity required, by gently challenging and creating new 'what if' possibilities and also the need to focus on the patient's/service users' and carers' viewpoints and experiences by actively using quotes and anecdotes from the survey and clinical experience (Element 5(ii) Applying knowledge and evidence).

Pat was also able to use knowledge and understanding of the requirements of the service and various organisations in order to align the goals, methods of working, recording, and producing data that fulfilled the obligations to account for service outcomes. Contributing this expertise to the planning process was valuable to the project and enabled simple but significant changes to be made which respected all the stakeholders and professions involved.

There were times in the process when Pat had to step up and challenge some difficult issues and attitudes by colleagues, some professional groups began by refusing to share information with colleagues in other sectors. The amount and nature of information about safety was a particular issue, some clinicians felt that support staff from the third sector should not be given details of safety concerns. Pat's personal approach was to challenge these notions, identify the duty of care everyone had to colleagues and bring the focus back to the people they all wanted to support, the patients/service users and carers. Pat tried to role model the transformation that they were seeking and motivate the group to achieve change, not in order to comply with guidance from the centre, but for the sake of the people they worked with.

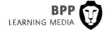

On a personal level, Pat showed respect for colleagues who had different views and ideas, the discussions were open, accepting and positive. Pat role modelled the belief that everyone had valuable ideas and comments; Pat brought the support staff, especially those from outside the statutory services, into the conversations and enabled them to voice their ideas. On one occasion a colleague stated that the views of the non-statutory services were irrelevant. Pat challenged this as incorrect, feeling that this did not reflect the values of the services or the needs of those receiving care. (Element 4(iii) Encouraging improvement). The initial statement had also conflicted with Pat's own values.

As the lead clinician for a service and team of staff, Pat also had a role in managing people (Element 3(iii) Managing people). When the changes in the process of assessing and recording information were finalised and agreed, Pat wrote the guidance and provided the support for team members as they piloted and then implemented the changes. One member of staff was struggling with the changes and felt that it was a lot of extra work for nothing; Pat provided extra supervision and support whilst the changes became more familiar and less effortful.

Nationally the process and outcome of the single assessment process for older adults was recognised as a blueprint for other services that need to provide integrated care across many agencies and professions. Pat has been able to showcase the learning from the experience in to other fields and teams. The local services have been able to build on the way the various teams and services worked together and have been able to provide a model of integrated care for a variety of client groups.

Case Study 3 Implementing radical service change

This case study aims to demonstrate how the CLCF can be used to develop, implement and evaluate new health care services or make changes to existing provision.

Over the last two decades there has been an emphasis on reducing the number of in-patient beds and transferring many aspects of acute care into the community setting. In part, this has been in response to the need to reduce burgeoning health care costs, but also due to the realisation that prolonged hospitalisation has a deleterious impact on the physical and psychological wellbeing of patients, particularly older people. In response to this there has been an increasing number of Hospital at Home (HaH) or Hospital Outreach Schemes developed in the UK to provide acute hospital level care in patients' own homes, either by facilitating early discharge following surgery, admission provision for people with chronic disease or end of life care (Jester, 2007).

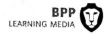

Specifically, HaH schemes have become increasingly used in trauma and orthopaedic settings to facilitate early discharge, typically reducing length of hospital stay in hospital following elective procedures such as total hip or knee replacement from 7 to 2 or 3 days. The efficacy of such schemes has been demonstrated in a growing body of literature (Jester & Hicks, 2003a & b; Siggeirsdottir et al; 2005; Mahomed et al; 2008).

Rebecca is an Advanced Nurse Practitioner in trauma and orthopaedics who led the development, implementation and evaluation of a number of HaH schemes to facilitate early discharge of patients following internal fixation of hip fracture and following elective procedures such as hip re-surfacing and replacement and knee replacement. This required Rebecca to have sound leadership competencies to plan and manage the resources (fiscal and human), team building and change management necessary to implement this type of service development.

The context of Rebecca's clinical practice requires her to exercise leadership across all 5 domains of the CLCF. Two of the domains, 'Domain 2: Working with others' and 'Domain 4: Improving services' were crucial to the implementation of the HaH.

Domain 2 Working with Others

Working with others comprises a number of competencies including, developing networks, building and managing relationships, encouraging contribution, working within teams. Rebecca invested in developing networks to ensuring that there was ownership of the idea of developing the HaH schemes from both the clinical teams within the acute hospital, the community based teams including GPs and the acceptability to patients and their families. From the outset she realised it was important to establish a steering group with representation from all the stakeholder groups and to not only present them with the rationale and evidence supporting the development of HaH, but to afford them the opportunity to raise their concerns and shape how the schemes would operate to minimise risk and optimise outcome. For example the GP and community nursing services were concerned that HaH would increase burden upon their services once patients were discharged to the scheme. To address these anxieties Rebecca arranged for a 24-hour helpline available 7 days per week as part of the new service and also provided assurance that medical responsibility for the patients remained with the orthopaedic consultant. She worked with the orthopaedic surgeons to help them understand that they would be able to retain overall medical responsibility for the patient, whilst knowing that nurses and physiotherapists from the orthopaedic unit would be providing the day to day care and treatment. Working with the steering group Rebecca was able to use her knowledge and skills to shape how the scheme would operate and also to influence the evaluation strategy, by determining what outcomes should be measured. She invited patient and family carer

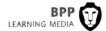

representatives onto the steering group to ensure their voice was heard and to reassure them that the degree of family burden was an important aspect of the evaluation.

Domain 4 Improving Services

The Improving services domain includes competence in:- ensuring patient safety, critically evaluating, encouraging improvement and innovation and facilitating transformation. All of these were required to ensure that the HaH schemes were at least as safe as traditional in-patient care. Rebecca worked with clinical colleagues to design and conduct pilots to persuade the hospital management of the value of HaH. As part of the pilots she worked with colleagues to evaluate the proposed new service, such as mortality, morbidity using both valid and reliable disease specific and generic quality of life measures, incidence of complications such as deep vein thrombosis, superficial wound infection, delayed deep sepsis, hip dislocation and pressure sores, carer burden using a valid carer burden index, length of stay, re-admission rates and psychometric measures of patient satisfaction. These data were collated as part of the pilot and compared to retrospective in-patient data to establish that HaH was as safe, effective and economical as the existing in-patient service.

To facilitate the necessary transformation from the existing to the new service Rebecca used the Improving Services domain of the CLCF to navigate the complexity of the changes required to shift from a current, more traditional, model of work practices where clinicians worked in silos to a more inter-disciplinary approach. She led on the training of nurses, physiotherapists and health care support workers to ensure their clinical knowledge, assessment and diagnostic skills were enhanced and that they felt equipped to transfer into a community based role, where they would be working without the ready support of colleagues as they had in the hospital.

Rebecca focussed on the benefits to the service users and argued the case for the nurses and physiotherapists to learn some of each other's skills. To minimise duplication of visits Rebecca was able to arrange for the physiotherapists to be trained in taking blood samples, giving sub-cutaneous injections and medication review. The nurses were given extra training in measuring range of joint movement, exercise regimes and teaching patients how to use various types of walking aids.

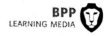

Case Study 4 A holistic review through a leadership lens

As healthcare professionals, paramedics are clinical leaders - utilising their knowledge, skills and experience to provide care and treatment for patients in environments and situations that are often challenging, complex and minimally resourced. This requires paramedics to make high quality decisions which are often time critical. The working environment is almost always unfamiliar, and the paramedic may be working alone or as part of a traditional two person ambulance crew. Often, the paramedic is the most senior clinician in attendance at calls for help and will have overall responsibility for patient care and decision-making. This includes leading and managing colleagues, co-ordinating resources and managing incident scenes. As such, paramedics have a significant impact, either directly or indirectly on the quality and safety of patient care, patient outcomes and experience.

Historically, the training and development of paramedics has focused upon the knowledge and technical skills required to provide appropriate care and treatment for patients, often in time critical and life threatening situations. It is only relatively recently; that a focus has started to be brought to the 'non-technical' or 'non-clinical' knowledge, skills and behaviours that are critical to the paramedic's role as a clinical leader, the effectiveness of the contribution that they can make – as individuals and collectively as a profession – to the process of clinical leadership.

The purpose of this case study is to raise awareness of the role paramedics have as clinical leaders, the contribution that they make to the process of clinical leadership and relate this to their day to day clinical practice, using the domains of the CLCF as the structure for the example.

Domain 1 Demonstrating Personal Qualities

Ahead of the start of a 12 hour day shift, the paramedic arrives at their designated ambulance station. The paramedic establishes which ambulance vehicle they are to work on for the shift, and learns that the colleague they are to work with for the day is a new student paramedic who they have not met or worked with before. Introductions are made and the paramedic provides the student with a quick tour of the ambulance station, with roles and responsibilities for the shift ahead being established. Together, the crew undertake pre-shift checks of the ambulance vehicle, equipment, drugs and supplies. The paramedic, having overall responsibility for the ambulance vehicle and patient care for the shift leads this checking process. The paramedic outlines the importance of the pre-shift checks to ensure patient and crew safety, ensures the student is familiar with the location of key pieces of equipment and shows the student where supplies and consumables are

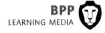

stored on the station. The importance of rectifying any shortages or defects found is re-enforced. The paramedic understands that they are a role model, and the importance of leading by example and setting high standards for others to follow.

Domain 2 Working with Others

The first 999 call that the crew are called to attend shortly after completing their pre-shift checks, is to a patient reported to be in cardiac arrest. On receipt of the call, the student paramedic informs his colleague that this will be the first cardiac arrest that they have attended. En-route to the call, the paramedic briefs the student about what they may expect, and also outlines the plan for how they will manage the incident upon arrival and what their expectations are of their colleague. As the senior clinician, the paramedic is responsible for assessing the incident scene, the patient and subsequently initiating treatment. The crew arrive at the incident. A volunteer Community First Responder (CFR) is already with the patient and has started basic life support. The paramedic re-assesses the situation and the patient – to ensure safety for all – and then formulates their action plan. The paramedic assumes the role of team leader and allocates tasks to others. Following best practice guidelines and established procedure, the paramedic considers that the resuscitation attempt has been unsuccessful. Prior to making the final decision to stop resuscitation and recognise the patient as 'life extinct', the paramedic asks the student paramedic for their opinion and feedback. The paramedic makes the decision to stop resuscitation, thanks the team for their efforts, and requests that his colleague inform the ambulance communications centre of the situation and request police attendance (to act as officers of the coroner). The paramedic then goes in to the next room to talk with the patient's relatives and inform them that the patient has died. After the incident, and en-route back to the ambulance station, the paramedic discusses the incident with the student. The paramedic is keen to gain feedback as to how the student felt the incident went, if anything could have been done differently, and what could be improved upon. Being aware that this was the first cardiac arrest that his colleague had attended, the paramedic recognises the importance of engaging the student in a de-brief and facilitating reflection on the incident to highlight any learning and areas for improvement to inform future practice.

Domain 3 Managing Services

The crew are called to attend reports of a Road Traffic Collision (RTC). Multiple vehicles are involved and it is reported that there are several patients. At the present time, they are the only ambulance crew in the area available to attend. The crew are the first emergency service vehicle to arrive at the scene.

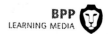

The principal priority of the paramedic is to assess the scene and ensure safety. Following initial scene assessment, the paramedic must determine how many patients are involved, how severely injured they are, and determine what additional resources are required. The paramedic provides the ambulance communications centre with an update. Having ensured scene safety, the paramedic then starts to further assess and treat the patient with severe injuries and who is trapped in one of the vehicles. The police and fire service arrive at the incident and take control of scene safety. As further ambulance service resources arrive, the paramedic provides a briefing as to the situation, the number of patients involved and an initial assessment of their injuries. The paramedic who was first on scene co-ordinates the subsequent resources that arrive. Due to the extent of his patient's injuries and the fact that they remain trapped, the paramedic requested the support of the air ambulance which carries an enhanced care team. The paramedic recognised that the patient would most likely benefit from this enhanced care being provided at the scene, and the air ambulance would enable the patient to be transported quickly to the major trauma centre for the region. This would enable less seriously injured patients to be transported by traditional ambulance to the nearby emergency department.

Domain 4 Improving Services

The next call received is to attend an elderly patient who has fallen in their home. Following thorough assessment, it is established that the fall was accidental, and that the patient has not sustained any injuries. The patient does not feel unwell, and does not wish to go to hospital. However, the patient lives alone and has no family or friends who live nearby. The house is cluttered, unclean and the crew notice that there are a number of potential 'trip' hazards that could result in the patient having another fall. The paramedic decides to gain the agreement of the patient to make a referral for them to the local falls prevention team, so that a thorough assessment can be made of their falls risk and to ascertain whether any measures can be put in place to prevent the patient falling again in future – which could result in injury. The paramedic also considers that the patient is vulnerable, and during conversation, the patient explains that they have been finding it increasingly difficult to look after themselves and their home. The paramedic gains consent to refer the patient to the local adult social services team for further assessment, and to see if any support can be put in place. The patient is happy that they do not have to go to hospital, as they feel safe in their own home. Reflecting on the incident on the way back to the ambulance station, the paramedic outlines for the student how important it is that paramedics have a focus upon preventing injury and disease from occurring in the first place. Often this can be achieved by making contact with primary and social care teams, and considering what could be done to improve a person's overall health and wellbeing.

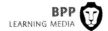

Domain 5 Setting Direction

Several of the calls responded to throughout the shift required the paramedic to utilise alternative care pathways for patients, as opposed to the default position being that all patients who needed to go to hospital were transported to the local emergency department. The major trauma patient from earlier in the shift was cared for, and managed, in accordance with the major trauma guideline which established criteria for those patients that should go directly to the major trauma centre and bypass the local emergency department. This is in response to a national change in practice, aimed at improving the quality of care, and outcomes for those experiencing major trauma. Similarly, the crew responded to a patient suffering from chest pains at one point in the shift. Following assessment, the paramedic decided that it was appropriate to transport the patient to a specialist cardiac centre – again bypassing the local emergency department, as all the evidence available suggests that the quality of patient care, and patient outcomes – across the healthcare system are improved by this approach. Similar arrangements are in place for patients who experience a stroke, and depending on outlined criteria, are known to do have better outcomes by being transported directly to hyper-acute stroke units.

In discussing these changes to the way in which patients are cared for by the local health system, and the changes this has required in terms of Paramedic clinical practice, the paramedic highlighted for the student that it was important to remember that such changes have come about as the result of evidence. Evidence suggests that certain patients, have better outcomes, depending on the type of treatment they receive and where they receive it. The impact of this change has been significant – not just for paramedic practice and the role of the ambulance service, but for all parts of the health system. The most important thing is that evidence based, best practice, should drive change and improvement. The role of the paramedic is to act as a role model in leading the implementation of changes in clinical practice that can have a positive impact on the quality of patient care, and their experience. Paramedics have an important role to play in participating in clinical audit projects to understand the implications that changes have had, and suggesting possible areas for further improvement and research.

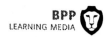

Chapter summary

- Improving the quality and safety of patient care requires clinical leadership.

- Clinical leadership can be regarded as a process.

- Clinicians as clinical leaders have a key role to play in raising the quality of the clinical leadership process – at individual, team, organisation, health system and professional levels.

- Acting as role models, leading by example, supporting the development of others and striving for excellence are key ways in which clinicians can contribute to clinical leadership.

- Clinicians must learn from experience and feedback, seeking out opportunities and challenges for learning and development.

- Clinical leadership is a shared responsibility – not limited to those who hold formal positions of management and leadership, but is a process that all healthcare professionals should be engaged with.

Three things to try

1. Access sources of information from inside and outside of the organisation, including patient feedback, to inform plans for service improvement.

2. Take part in multi-agency case conferences and share the learning by de-briefing colleagues.

3. Set up a local clinical network to facilitate greater cooperation across the health economy.

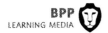

Chapter references

Jester, R, and Hicks, C. Using cost-effectiveness analysis to compare hospital at home and in-patient interventions. *Part 1. Journal of Clinical Nursing 2003; 12.13–19.*

Jester, R, and Hicks, C. Using cost-effectiveness analysis to compare hospital at home and in-patient interventions. *Part 2 Journal of Clinical Nursing 2003; 12.20–27.*

Jester R (2007). *Advancing Practice in Rehabilitation Nursing.* Blackwell Publishing. Oxford.

Goodwin, N, Smith, J, Davies, A, Perry, C, Rosen, R, Dixon, A, Dixon, J and Ham, C (2011) *Integrated care for patients and populations: Improving outcomes by working together.* London: The Kings Fund.

Kodner, D, Spreeuwenberg, C. Integrated Care: Meaning, logic, applications, and implications – a discussion paper. *International Journal of Integrated Care 2002; (2). [Online]* Available at: www.ijic.org/index.php/ijic/article/view/67 [Accessed 13 November 2012].

Mahomed N N, Davis A, M, Hawker, G, Badley, E, Davey J, R, Syed K, A, Coyte P, C, Gandhi R, Wright J, G Inpatient compared with home-based rehabilitation following primary unilateral total hip or knee replacement: a randomized controlled trial. *The Journal of bone and joint surgery 2008; American 90 (8) 1673–80*

Royal Pharmaceutical Society (2011) Leadership competency Framework for pharmacy professionals. *Royal Pharmaceutical Society,* London.

NHS Improving Quality (2013) NHS IQ [Online] Available at www.england.nhs.uk

Siggeirsdottir K, Olafsson O, Jonsson H, Iwarsson S, Gudnason V, AU: Jonsson J. Short hospital stay augmented with education and home-based rehabilitation improves function and quality of life after hip replacement: randomized study of 50 patients with 6 months of follow-up. *Acta orthopaedica 2005; 76 (4) 555–62.*

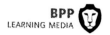

Chapter 10

Learning leadership in a clinic or service setting

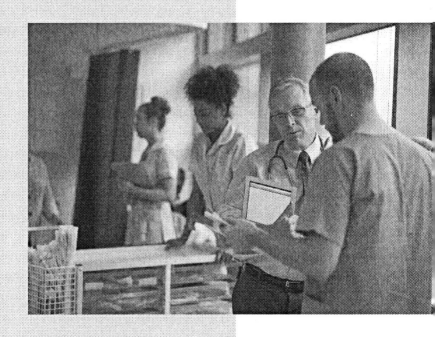

Learning leadership in a clinic or service setting

Chapter overview

This chapter provides:

- A description of the 5 domains of the CLCF and how they relate to a clinic or service setting

- Four case studies describing leadership in practice

Introduction

Within a clinic or service setting nurses and allied health professionals experience a greater degree of autonomy. There has been a plethora of nurse-led clinics established across many clinical conditions in recent years. Clinicians have their own case load and can make the decision to discharge the patient or refer to other more appropriate healthcare colleagues based on their own assessment (Hatchett, 2003). This freedom, whilst bringing with it greater responsibility and accountability for the clinician, also requires a more strategic leader with greater awareness not only of themselves but also the environment in which they operate both internal and external to the organisation.

Clinics established by nursing and allied health professionals offer patients greater choice and are usually designed around the patient for improved flexibility and accessibility. They have been endorsed by the Department of Health as a way to speed up access to specialist healthcare. Measuring effectiveness should be an integral part of the service and should encompass both audit and evaluation. Clinical audit has been defined by NICE (2002) as *'A quality improvement process that seeks to improve patient care and outcomes through systematic review of care against explicit criteria and the implementation of change'* thus promoting a culture of continuous improvement.

Demonstrating Personal Qualities

In a clinic setting clinicians are often working autonomously, hence the setting provides a rich environment to develop leadership

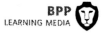

qualities. Continuing professional development is critical in this environment to maintain credibility with other colleagues and patients as they are often working in highly specialised areas with a greater decision-making role. The features of this domain: managing self, acting with integrity and self-awareness are key leadership qualities when spearheading a service and managing a patient caseload. The outpatient setting is ideal to gain patient feedback on their experience of the service and recommendations for improvement.

Working with Others

Establishing a successful clinic often requires the need to collaborate with other clinical and non-clinical staff. Understanding and appreciating how a service impacts on others within the outpatient department and the role that they play in ensuring the service is successful helps to build relationships and ensure sustainability. The roles within the outpatient department are many and varied ranging from administrative and clerical staff and porters to clinical staff such as doctors, other allied professionals and pathology departments. Often the establishment and maintenance of a clinic requires collaboration with senior management in the organisation and commissioners, it is necessary to develop this network of colleagues to foster success and ensure a quality experience for patients.

Managing Services

Ensuring the clinic is cost effective and provides value for money is also essential to its longevity. Managing resources is central to this, ensuring the right person is doing the right thing in the right place at the right time every time improves efficiency. There are additional elements to an outpatient service which require management these include improving Did Not Attend (DNA) rates, capturing activity and analysing the impact of the clinic on patient outcomes and experience. The cost of a missed appointment is approximately £100, annually this accrues to £600 million, initiatives such as telephone or text message reminders have had an impact in this area. Capturing activity and performance data is crucial particularly for correct remuneration via payment by results (PbR) and resource management however effective systems need to be developed to collect such data.

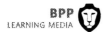

Improving Services

When looking to improve outpatient services discussion and feedback with all those mentioned previously including patients can help to drive through ideas for improvement. Implementing a tool to obtain patient and carer feedback is a useful method for identifying areas for improvement (Wensing *et al*; 2003). It is also important to demonstrate to patients that their opinions have been listened to and acted upon. There are many tools available in healthcare now to obtain user views some are web-based or portable touch screen devices, but all should be seen as a tool for quality improvement.

Setting Direction

As described in other chapters the NHS is undergoing significant change and new patient pathways are evolving, this gives impetus to try something different in the outpatient setting. Access for many patients can be an issue whether that is because of geographical distance to the hospital and problems with transport or age making travel challenging, delivering outpatient services in the community can be the answer to some of these issues. For those working in outpatients it is worth considering your target audience and whether there are solutions to access problems.

Case Study 1 If you have a vision, you too can change the service

Domain 5 Setting Direction

Paula is a consultant midwife involved in the development of a new purpose-built midwifery led Birth Centre (BC) in response to a national drive to promote normal birth (Royal College of Midwives, 2000). In approaching the task she used the CLCF to reflect on how it could help her do this well.

Applying her knowledge (Element 5(ii)) she was confident that the physical attributes of the BC, such as a homely, relaxing environment would support normal birth. Using evidence (Element 5(ii)) Paula had read some research which showed that the environment alone would not guarantee that physiological birth would be protected and that routine midwifery care sometimes resulted in unnecessary intervention (Clarke & Bowcock, 2003;

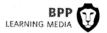

BJM, 2011; Clarke et al; 2007). She acknowledged that the close proximity of the large obstetric unit next door has advantages should a problem occur but that the proximity of the medical facilities led some sceptics to question how care at the new BC would differ from the traditional model.

Domain 1 Demonstrating Personal Qualities

As the senior responsible clinician and project lead with a significant amount of experience Paula decided to initiate a review of the care provided for women anticipating a normal birth. She chose the development of an Integrated Care Pathway (ICP) as the approach to assist with supporting and protecting physiological birth at the new service. As the new service impacted on a large cross section of staff Paula role modelled leadership behaviours through being considerate to the concerns of her colleagues and seeking to gain consensus for the project.

Domain 2 Working with Others

Numerous people were involved with the change and included: the head of clinical governance; care pathway facilitator, librarian and more than 100 midwives. Paula invested considerable time talking to and addressing queries from midwives. She organised meetings to raise awareness and invited doctors, midwives and other interested staff and service users using flyers and emails. Recognising that clinicians are busy people and wanting to get the maximum attendance Paula arranged to hold the meetings at time when most staff were available.

Paula was aware that the project would be more successful if she gained the buy-in from senior midwives, the medical director, obstetricians and the consultant lead for clinical risk. Paula established a project team and used the development of the ICP as the catalyst for junior and senior clinicians to work together. Recognising the importance of involving the service user the ICP was also developed in collaboration with women.

Midwives with an appreciation of evidence-based practice volunteered to review specific areas of practice and brought their findings to the group. Junior midwives utilised their recently completed assignment work and student midwives and medical students also participated. Everyone's view and contribution was respected and considered for inclusion. The trust clinical librarian provided appraisal of the relevant literature. Where evidence was absent or equivocal, expert consensus was achieved by actively seeking the views of others, from sources within and outside the Trust.

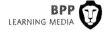

Domain 4 Improving Services

By anticipating and minimising potential risk, every aspect of care was considered to ensure the ICP would support and guide staff to deliver consistently safe clinical practice and high quality care, which was ratified by the Trust's solicitors (Element 4(i) Ensuring patient safety).

During development, the ICP was piloted (Element 4(ii) Critically evaluating). Student midwives used it in parallel with a midwife using traditional records. This exercise was to demonstrate that the same account of events could be recreated and ensure the ICP captured key aspects of care. It was acknowledged that the initial version of the ICP would not be perfect and recognised it would provide a tool for continuous assessment and improvement. Women and staff were encouraged to provide verbal and written feedback with suggestions for change. Regular ICP meetings continued and were used to discuss recommendations for change and agreement for version two. Paula and the project team undertook an audit which revealed encouraging improvements:

- Increased variety of birth positions – from 20% (Peters 2003) to 68%

- Increased use of water for labour and birth – 1% to 13%

- Increase of physiological third stage – negligible numbers to 27%

- Women going home directly from the BC – from negligible numbers initially to 37%

Domain 3 Managing Services

The enormity of the task of developing an ICP should not be underestimated. It took a significant amount of planning and resources, such as time, commitment from the team and motivation to achieve the goal. Acting as a lead champion was important as Paula involved all the staff involved in providing care. The project team used an audit to subsequently demonstrate that the ICP was not only instrumental in improving care from the outset, but that improvements to the service have not only been sustained but also enhanced further.

The ICP has evolved significantly since its development. It has subsequently been updated in line with new evidence and now also incorporates Clinical Negligence for Trust (CNST) standards. From the outset, the ICP was developed with the intention of it being suitable for electronic use. The ICP has been incorporated into electronic documentation for labour and birth. The company who has incorporated the ICP electronically are promoting its use for birth centres nationally.

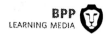

Case Study 2 Promoting better health and outcomes

This case study discusses development made by a Clinical Nurse Specialist (CNS) in Limb Reconstruction working within a large city teaching hospital. The CNS regularly assessed patients both before and after their surgery and it became clear that health promotion messages regarding smoking cessation preoperatively were not having the desired effect of even a small number of patients quitting the habit before their admission. In taking steps to address the shortcomings in health promotion identified, the CNS was able to show how the CLCF can guide action. This case study in particular illustrates leadership particularly in the following Domains; 2 Working with Others, Domain 4 Improving Services and Domain 5 Setting Direction.

The role of the CNS preoperatively was largely to counsel and prepare patients for what was often lengthy treatment and help them to optimise their recovery. It was clear a large cohort of the preoperative patients were smokers, an activity that is known to have grave consequences for general health but that can also impact negatively on both wound and bone healing and subsequently the whole limb reconstruction process. On speaking to patients already receiving treatment post operatively, whilst they had been advised to stop smoking, the CNS discovered that patients did not fully appreciate the harmful impact of smoking on the reconstruction of their limb, nor had they been directed to support they could access to help them take the necessary steps to quit, either before or after their surgery (Element 4(ii) Critically evaluating, 5(i) Identifying the contexts for change). It appeared that some junior staff involved in the preoperative care of these patients were ill equipped to deliver this vital health promotion message so improvements were urgently required (Element 4(i) Ensuring patient safety, 4(iii) Encouraging improvement). Other clinics within the hospital were visited by the CNS to assess the resources they used for smoking cessation as well as internet searches into how other hospital trusts manage the problem (Element 5(ii) Applying knowledge and evidence).

Research and literature on the effects of smoking on bone and wound healing, particularly in limb reconstruction situations were explored by the CNS, and other closely related specialities who either had input with limb reconstruction patients or who may have found any results relevant to their own clinical practice were approached (Element 2(i) Building and maintain relationships). Research showed that a combination of both stop smoking literature and follow up support was required (Element 4(iv) Innovation and facilitating transformation). It also became clear that to address the apparent shortcomings in health promotion messages being given across some specialities a collaborative approach was required (Element 2(i) Developing networks). Discussions were had between

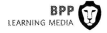

the appropriate specialities to gain different perspectives on the issue (Element 2(ii) Building and maintaining relationships, Element 4(iv) Innovation and facilitating transformation) as well as to encourage contribution from a wider field of professionals (Element 2(iii) Encouraging contribution) and ensure any resulting patient literature was fit for purpose across different clinical teams (Element 2(iv) Working within teams). The importance of regular communication between these teams was not underestimated and the CNS realised the importance of engaging all those involved to make certain that teams were on board in order for the planned change to be implemented effectively (Element 2(iii) Encouraging contribution, Element 4(iii) Encouraging improvement, Element 4(iv) Innovation and facilitating transformation).

The CNS then focussed on, and took the lead in, devising a patient information leaflet to be used across four different specialities who had become involved (Element 2(iv) Working within teams). Initially the leaflet was piloted across two clinics to gain both patient and clinical teams' feedback (Element 4(ii) Critically evaluating). Initially the leaflet took the shape of a patient fact sheet using the 'Stop Before Your Op' campaign that other trusts had successfully run elsewhere (Element 5(ii) Applying knowledge and evidence). It was clear to the CNS that the change needed to be both sustained and developed however (Element 5(iv) Evaluating impact). To this end, following the pilot period and a successful evaluation the information sheet was submitted to the trust Communications Department to be developed into a trust wide leaflet with a request to launch a hospital wide 'Stop Before Your Op' campaign for all pre-operative patients, in any specialty (Element 4(iv) Innovation and facilitating transformation, Element 2(i) Developing networks). As a result, a plan was formulated between the CNS and the Communications team to make the Stop Before Your Op patient information available to all staff on the intranet and a paragraph regarding smoking cessation and the support available to patients to be included on all future patient information leaflets. This could therefore assist any patients who may be persuaded to give up smoking and would provide the support that they need to quit. Overall the goal of attempting to enhance patient safety and improve recovery following any surgery through improvements in smoking cessation advice was achieved (Element 5(iv) Evaluating impact). The seed of a vision for the future of smoking cessation within the organisation was also sewn, with improvements in health promotion reflecting the core values of the NHS as a whole.

The CNS felt it was vital they did not lose sight of the importance of team working and collaboration in bringing about a positive change for both patients and the service as a whole however (Element 2(iv) Working within teams, Element 4(iii) Encouraging improvement, Element 4(iv) Innovation and facilitating transformation). The next fundamental stage to the project recognised by the CNS was that of succession planning in order to sustain both the change implemented and the potential improvement in patient safety and recovery

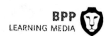

(Element 5(iv) Evaluating impact, Element 4(iii) Encouraging improvement, Element 4(iv) Innovation and facilitating transformation). In this case the CNS concluded that there was a requirement for more emphasis to be placed on smoking cessation at every stage in the patient journey, either by all clinical staff working closer with existing health promotion and addiction services, or by regional and local NHS based resources being more widely used within the trust (Element 2(i) Developing networks, Element 2(ii) Building and maintaining relationships).

This case study begins to provide the CNS with further ideas on how smoking cessation could be developed in the future and suggests that further work needs to be carried out, perhaps formulating plans for how others could be motivated to work towards achieving the shared vision of better health promotion and healthier patients both before and after surgery of all kinds.

Case Study 3 Developing me, whilst supporting others: the power of personal reflection

As part of a COPD team working across four Trusts, Millie had responsibility for the development of an existing pulmonary rehabilitation (PR) service running in both primary and secondary care. The main objective was to evaluate and improve the efficiency and capacity of the service to accommodate increasing demand, whilst improving quality and effectiveness. Millie identified that the assessment process for PR presented an opportunity for transformation. The following case study outlines the transformation that took place with reference to the CLCF Domain 2 Working with Others, Domain 4 Improving Services and Domain 5 Setting Direction. This case study also illustrates how clinical leadership activities can be carried out by healthcare professionals who do not occupy formal leadership positions and how the CLCF can be used to support staff at all levels with service development.

The PR assessment clinics in secondary care were multi-disciplinary and included a respiratory consultant physician who oversaw, and held ultimate responsibility for the PR service. All patients were seen by the consultant who made the final decision regarding acceptance onto the programme. Millie identified this as a potentially inefficient use of resources and unnecessary step in the pathway for the majority of attendees given that most were already known to a respiratory specialist; be it physician, specialist GP or COPD Team (Element 3(ii) Managing resources). Additionally, the physiotherapy staff in the clinic had specialist knowledge and skills in the management of COPD and delivery of PR. These staff were well positioned to make autonomous decisions

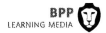

regarding patient suitability for PR. Other issues included; long wait times in clinic for the consultant, inability to establish additional clinics due to lack of consultant availability, a six month waiting list and lack of engagement with local under-utilised community PR programmes. Demand for PR was projected to increase further as a result of primary care COPD initiatives.

Millie recognised several barriers to the potential transformation. The PR service in secondary care was well established and run by healthcare professionals more senior in grade than Millie. That, combined with the consultant-led professional hierarchy of power inherent within the organisational culture, presented a challenge when instigating change. Millie acknowledged that the threat of change was likely to induce apprehension and resistance, particularly because she was new and unknown within the team.

Millie recognised that building and maintaining effective working relationships with her new colleagues was fundamental (Element 2(ii) Building and maintaining relationships) if she was to successfully mobilise the staff to review current practice and challenge the status quo (Element 4(iii) Encouraging improvement). Development of networks (Element 2(i) Developing networks) was also vital for eliciting change. Key stakeholders, including the consultant, were prompted to engage in dialogue and debate, critically evaluate the service (Element 4(ii) Critically evaluating) and reach consensus regarding objectives and action plans (Element 5(iii) Making decisions). Such networks enabled collaborative working within both the PR and wider COPD teams (Element 2(iv) Working within teams) and the opportunity to establish relationships and mutual respect. Millie understood the importance of encouraging contribution from all involved in the PR service (Element 2(iii) Encouraging contribution) to enable colleagues to have ownership of any service change. Consideration of others' needs, views and expertise was important, as was creating a tolerant, listening environment to avert any feelings of threat. Taking time to invest in relationships before suggesting change, alongside demonstrating personal integrity, (Element 1(iv) Acting with integrity) was crucial for Millie to gain the trust, support and followership of her new colleagues (Element 2(ii) Building and maintaining relationships).

Over 18 months, Millie facilitated transformation of the service through evaluation and gradual pathway re-design (Element 4(iv) Innovation and facilitating transformation). She encouraged dialogue within and across the primary/secondary care interface to bring about creative solutions to problems identified in the patient pathway (Element 4(iii) Encouraging improvement). Patient safety was at the core of the transformation, the effect of any proposed change on service users being risk assessed throughout (Element 4(i) Ensuring patient safety). As part of a multi-system COPD Team, Millie was responsible for promoting the wider context for change to front-line clinicians (Element 5(i)

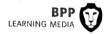

Identifying contexts for change), for example the need to shift care closer to the patient, establish equal access and patient choice within the PR service, and align with the QIPP model. Once relationship and trust had been established, Millie was able to apply her specialist PR knowledge and experience in conjunction with evidence to challenge existing practices and processes and influence key players including the consultant (Element 5(ii) Applying knowledge and evidence). Millie undertook robust evaluation throughout the transformation to demonstrate and communicate the impact of the service changes on users and providers (Element 5(iv) Evaluating impact).

Despite not having any formal authority Millie demonstrated leadership behaviour and several aspects of the PR assessment process were successfully transformed for the benefit of users and providers. Management of the assessment process was handed over to the physiotherapy and occupational therapy professionals, who now lead the clinics with on-site access to a respiratory registrar for medical support. Responsibility for clinical decisions regarding patients' suitability for PR lies with the therapists who now run additional autonomous clinics to increase assessment capacity. Prior to assessment, referrals are now triaged according to clinical need and patient location, selecting the most appropriate PR programme in primary or secondary care. All patients are offered choice regarding the programme they attend and are able to move between sites at any point along their PR journey. This flexibility has led to increased activity at community sites and a reduced waiting list for the programme in secondary from 6 months to 4-8 weeks. Utilising networks to ensure collaborative working strengthened links between PR staff working in both primary and secondary care, promoting effective communication between teams to secure a seamless service for all patients referred to the service.

Millie reflected on her personal learning throughout the process (Element 1(iii) Continuing professional development), both independently and through joint discussion with her line manager. Key personal learning points were identified as follows: effective implementation of change within a well-established culture takes time and may best be achieved through gradual, incremental steps; relationship is of absolute importance in influencing attitudes and behaviour; healthcare professionals who do not occupy a formal leadership position can effectively undertake leadership activities and are often well placed to identify opportunities for change at the front-line; and networks provide an effective way to engage and promote collaborative working within and between teams. Millie plans to continue to refer to the CLCF self-assessment tool to identify ongoing development needs and facilitate her progress as an effective clinical leader.

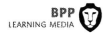

Chapter summary

In this chapter we learned:

- Working in a clinic setting provides a rich environment to develop leadership qualities due to the greater responsibility and accountability for the clinician.

- Clinicians require a greater awareness not only of themselves but also the environment in which they operate both internal and external to the organisation.

- This highlights the importance of with working across organisational boundaries both within and outside the clinic and the need to identifying best possible solutions for their patients.

- The outpatient setting is ideal to gain patient feedback on their experience of the service and recommendations for improvement.

Three things to try

1. Take the lead in a multi-disciplinary team meeting to review a clinical case.

2. Act as a mentor to students and peers faced with difficult ethical judgments.

3. Use audit outcomes to challenge current practice and develop consistent, reliable care.

Chapter references

Birthplace in England Collaborative group. Perinatal and maternal outcomes by planned place of birth for healthy women with low risk pregnancies: the Birthplace in England national prospective cohort study. *British Journal of Midwifery 2011; 343:d7400. 1–13.*

Campbell, H, Hotchkiss, R, Bradshaw, N, Porteous, M (1998) Integrated Care Pathways *British Medical Journal 1998; (316) 133–137.*

Clarke, P, Bowcock, M (2003) Audit of Midwifery Led Care and observations. *Birmingham Women's Health Care NHS Trust.*

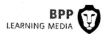

Clarke, P, Bowcock, M, Gales, P. Development of an integrated care pathway for natural birth. *British Journal Midwifery 2007; (15) 1.*

De Luc, K, Currie, L. (1999) Developing, Implementing and Evaluating Care Pathways in the UK: The Way to Go. *HSMC Research Report* The University of Birmingham, ISBN0704421089.

Docherty, B, McCombe, J, Simpson, S. Protocol-based care: 2. Developing pathways with effective teams *Professional Nurse 2003; 19 (2) 97–101.*

Hatchett, R (2003) *Nurse-led Clinics: Practice Issues.* London: Routledge.

Peters,E (2003). Audit of 'Positions adopted for birth. *Birmingham Women's NHS Health Care Trust.* (Unpublished). Birmingham.

Royal College of Midwives (2000) *Vision 2000* Royal College of Midwives. London.

Wensing, M, Vingerhoets, E and Grol, R. Feedback based on patient evaluations: a tool for quality improvement? *Patient Education and Counselling* 2003; 51(2):149–53.

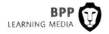

Chapter 10

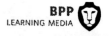

Chapter 11

Supporting leadership learning – tutor notes

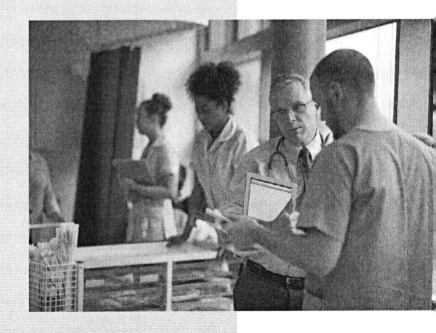

Supporting leadership learning – tutor notes

Chapter overview

This chapter provides:

- A description of leadership and continuous learning.
- The importance of insight, feedback and review.
- Tools and techniques for assessment.

Introduction

The CLCF can be used by health and care organisations, professional bodies, educators and individuals to:

- Help with personal development planning and career progression.
- Help with the design and commissioning of formal training curricula and development programmes by colleges and societies, higher education institutions, and public healthcare providers.
- Highlight individual strengths and development areas through self-assessment, appraisal and structured feedback from colleagues.

Previous chapters have focused on leadership learning in different career stages – pre and post qualifying, and clinical settings – acute/ward and community/primary care. The concepts discussed have been written for the individual, either a clinician or supervisor, and provide useful concepts, tools and techniques as they seek to develop their understanding and experience in leadership and management.

For clinicians undertaking formal education and training their courses will cover a broad range of topics. It is important that leadership learning is incorporated within the mainstream curriculum, rather than regarded as something additional or even peripheral to that core.

For colleagues working in higher education institutions or in workplace training facilities there is guidance to assist with

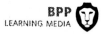

integrating the CLCF into education and training. The *Guidance for Integrating the Clinical Leadership Competency Framework into Education and Training* describes the knowledge, skills, attitudes and behaviours required for each domain and provides suggestions for appropriate learning and development activities to be delivered throughout education and training, as well as possible methods of assessment. The scenarios used as examples will be invaluable to health faculties and clinical students, and will stimulate novel special study components which will further enhance leadership skills.

In this final chapter we are changing the emphasis to provide a tutor's or trainer's perspective on leadership development. Building on the individual ideas from previous chapters, we will focus on broader concepts and organizational challenges with the aim of supporting trainers to develop work-based, experiential programmes of leadership learning within their workplace.

Feedback to support learning – providing insight

The training process in almost any sphere one can think of involves feedback. In the acquisition of clinical skills trainees will receive feedback from a more experienced colleague on how they have undertaken a procedure or dealt with a patient. We advocate a position whereby feedback about the use of leadership competencies is integrated with that of the acquisition of clinical skills such that the processes become indivisible. In this way the use of leadership competencies become part of normal practice and importantly leadership is 'normalised' rather than separated from clinical practice. The learner needs feedback, but developmental feedback, so that it can be used to change or improve some aspect of their work behaviour. King (1999) suggests that giving feedback is not just to provide a judgment or evaluation. It is to provide insight. The 'insight' gained helps the student understand their own strengths and weaknesses. Thus for the tutor the key skills are to listen and ask, not, as is often the temptation, to tell and provide solutions (King, 1999).

The concept of insight or self-awareness is a central element of leadership and a core element of the CLCF – Demonstrating

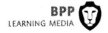

Personal Qualities. Using feedback methods to help learners to gain insight and develop their own self-awareness is extremely important for trainers to work on.

Approaches to using feedback to support learning

An approach widely used in the NHS since the early 1990s is often referred to as Pendletons Rule's. This approach focuses on encouraging the person receiving the feedback, the learner, to give their reflections on their own performance and with an emphasis on placing positive comments alongside development feedback.

1. The learner states what was done well.

2. The observer states what was done well.

3. The learner states what could be improved.

4. The observer states what could be improved, and *how* this might be done.

However, this method of feedback has come under criticism for being too rigid, formulaic and predictable. Many learners become so familiar with the method that there is a lack of meaningful discussion, and much of the 'what can be improved' section of discussion, are dressed up as being developmental, with the common perception being 'this is the time for negative criticism to come my way' (Spurgeon & Klaber, 2011). The end result is that the feedback may not lead to genuine insight or actual change.

Perhaps a method more conducive to leadership development is one that educationalists call a 'narrative approach'. This approach builds on Pendleton's concepts and is where the learner and observer work together in a chronological way to recall and reflect on what happened step-by-step, teasing out learning points along the way. If well facilitated, this can be a very constructive approach and the observations and comments of other observers can be included to enrich the feedback.

Another approach is what is called an agenda led, outcomes based analysis (Silverman *et al*; 1996). In this method, the observer starts with the learner's agenda by asking them what problems they have experienced and what help they would like from you

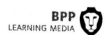

and any other observers who might be present (Silverman cited in Spurgeon & Klaber, 2011). This is done by encouraging self-assessment and problem solving before you, and eventually the whole group, contribute to problem solving. Feedback should be descriptive, balanced and objective and the person giving feedback must avoid sounding judgmental.

Dr Bob Klaber *et al* (2012) in a companion book to this text aimed at medical colleagues provide a number of helpful advice about giving feedback in a wide range of contexts:

- **Be learner led:** ask the learner how they would most like to receive feedback; if they don't have a particular view then give them two or three options which have worked well for others previously. Ensure the discussions are interactive and keep returning to the learner's self-perceptions and agenda.

- **Be flexible:** a successful facilitator/training will have several different techniques they feel comfortable using to deliver feedback. Being adaptable and responsive in real-time to whether or not different approaches are working is crucial.

- **Focus on achieving outcomes/improvement/change:** whatever strategies you adopt, it is important to focus on supporting the learner to continually seek improvement, however impressive their performance is. One of the definitions of excellence is a relentless desire to improve. Summarising with emphasis on outcomes and how to achieve improvements can be helpful.

- **Structure is important, but avoid being predictable:** much of the literature on feedback is focused on the importance of being structured and while this is important, if the learner is only half listening to the positive feedback as they wait for imminent negatives, there is little gained. This is a particular problem with the feedback sandwich where positive feedback is positioned either side of an area for improvement.

- **Be descriptive, balanced and objective:** where possible, providing descriptive examples can help a learner to recall and reflect on particular issues. Being objective, balanced and focused on behaviours rather than becoming personal gives the process the feeling of being supportive and fair – it is extremely important for learners to feel positive about the feedback experience, even if there is much to work on, so they can go on to effect change.

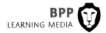

- **Take opportunities to feedback in different time frames:** although some learning opportunities are one-off episodes, ideally trainers should look to establish a strong relationship with learners where feedback can be given, and worked on, longitudinally in time. This approach is much more developmental and can offset that difficult dilemma, after observing a particularly problematic episode, about how much feedback one learner can receive in a single sitting.

- **Relate to principles, concepts and evidence:** if the opportunity arises, relating specific feedback points to wider concepts and evidence can be a useful way of conceptualising them. This is a helpful technique to depersonalize and broaden the ideas presented.

- **Don't hide from difficult feedback:** this is one area rarely mentioned in the feedback literature, despite being an area of significant concern for many trainers. As a trainer it can be at times uncomfortable, vulnerable and risky contemplating highlighting problematic issues with a learner. In many ways this is similar experience to how you approach difficult conversations with patients, where preparation is key.

The ideas discussed above will help facilitate a development process which is achievable. It is crucial that, at some stage, appropriate feedback is given, as otherwise the learner will have no chance of gaining the insight needed to develop as a leader.

Tools

Self-assessment

By reading the CLCF any clinician may be able to assess their leadership behaviours across the five domains of the framework. To assist with personal development there is also a self-assessment tool to help individuals identify where their leadership strengths and development needs lie. Consisting of a short questionnaire for each domain, the self-assessment tool uses a three point Likert scale to rate how often a statement applies to you. Users can then tally up their scores to identify leadership behaviours that may be under or overplayed, thus allowing them to manage their own learning and development by allowing reflection on which areas of the CLCF they would like to develop further.

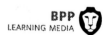

Having completed the self-assessment, we would encourage individuals to discuss their results with their line manager, mentor or trusted colleague. Individuals may find it helpful to ask their line manager or colleagues to also download the document and rate the individual against some or all of the leadership domains. Coming together and comparing the ratings with the individual's self-ratings can provide valuable insight into their leadership behaviour. For example, students or colleagues working in pairs, then three, then small groups may rate themselves and each other to facilitate a learning experience using the self-assessment tool.

The NHS Leadership Academy online self-assessment tool is linked to a personal action plan template to help individuals consolidate their development areas.

360° Feedback

360° feedback is a powerful tool to help individuals identify where their leadership strengths and development needs lie. The process includes getting confidential feedback from line managers, peers and direct reports. As a result, it gives an individual an insight into other people's perceptions of their leadership abilities and behaviour.

The 360° technique involves the systematic collection of performance data on an individual, gathered from a variety of sources called raters. The raters normally include the participant's line manager, peers and direct reports. It can also involve others individuals, who may not be peers or direct reports, but who are people the participant still works with closely with, or colleagues from other organisations. The choice of raters in any particular case tend to include those who have had enough regular contact with the participant to be able to observe and assess his/her behaviours at work. Because each rater offers a different perspective on the participant's skills and abilities, the resulting appraisal provides a well-rounded and complete picture of the participant and his/her strengths and weaknesses in assessed areas.

The 360° technique is always confidential and it is recommended to use a minimum of three raters, so that their anonymity can be assured and that they can feel to provide open and honest observations. In industry 360° feedback can be undertaken by simply emailing colleagues and asking them to send feedback or

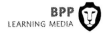

observations about an individual to their line manager. In the NHS it is recommended to use a more structured tool where the data is collected using an online process, where a written report on the raters' collated observations is provided to the participant as part of a feedback session by a qualified facilitator.

Online learning

Many students are familiar with working online. There is an excellent e-learning resource available on the National Learning Management System called LeAD which is appropriate for all clinical staff regardless of profession, specialty, or stage of training and offers one component of an overall leadership training and development programme.

LeAD reflects the leadership competences outlined in the CLCF and has 50 short e-learning sessions that will help clinicians develop the knowledge, skills, attitudes and behaviours through inter-active sessions which the learner can progress through.

Each session is designed to stand alone in order to provide an open learning pathway to meet individual development needs and interests and higher education institutions may use LeAd as an online component of a pre or post registration course. For example, the Centre for Postgraduate Pharmacy Education (CPPE) has integrated LeAD into Supporting Leadership Series which includes pre and post activities and a series of self-directed modules run over 12 months.

Workplace learning

When clinicians enter the workforce the CLCF can be used or adapted to help with professional development, such as continuing professional development (CPD), required or provided by their employer, society or college.

These may include undertaking audits or service improvement projects using methods such as the PDSA cycles in Chapter 7. Many of the learning and development opportunities identified in the CLCF at student and practitioner level apply equally at practitioner or experienced practitioner level. The learning opportunities such as seeking opportunities to learn from other professionals in everyday practice or through formal opportunities - collaborating

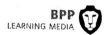

with or shadowing other colleagues, obtaining patients views - are consistent with good care provision, emphasising the leadership as an integrated, rather than separate, set of behaviours. Case Study 1 in Chapter 9 illustrates how the practitioner, used the learning and development activity within the CLCF to structure her development over 12 months.

Case Study Element 2(ii): Building and maintaining relationships

The lead educator for a qualifying programme in occupational therapy, identified the need and value of strengthening local manager/clinical input to his programme's development and delivery. He organised an initial one-day workshop session at the start of the programme review process, with the aim of promoting debate and discussion on changing service needs, exploring how these should inform development of the programme, and teasing out and addressing initial queries and concerns regarding significant change to the existing programme. She wanted to ensure a sharing of perspectives and to enable a full contribution from the outset of the review process from colleagues whose support for different ways of structuring and delivering the programme would be crucial. In this way, she built up trust and a genuinely collaborative approach to the new programme's development, paving the way for a successful revalidation/re-approval.

Dynamic learning environments, using service improvement techniques and action learning

Creating environments for learners that promote the opportunity for them to develop and learn is crucial. Most employing bodies invest a sizeable amount in workplace training and education aimed at improving quality of care. While a lot of this activity is focused on technical aspects of practice, there is often also development activity, which is suitable for leadership development.

Techniques that are used in the workplace as leadership development opportunities include lean methods, such as value stream mapping. Lean thinking is basically about getting the right things in the right place, at the right time, in the right quantities, while minimizing waste and being open and flexible to change and as such provide useful environments for leadership behaviours to be modelled.

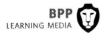

For leaders handling complex improvement challenges a popular learning method involves a group of people, usually peers with similar roles or levels of responsibilities, meeting regularly over a set period of time, normally 12-15 months. The group known as a set, contract with each other to meet 5 or 6 times through this period and agree to follow established ground rules to participate in a facilitated discussion involving reflected learning and action. An action learning set can be in-house with peers from your organisation or a cross sector set for leaders which bring together top level staff from different sectors and professional backgrounds (Revans, 1976).

Action Learning Sets (ALS) can use a trained facilitator or may choose to facilitate the process themselves.

ALS are widely used throughout the NHS to promote leadership development because they provide the opportunity to work on real problems by creating the space for leaders to learn from each other. They can be combined with workshops, mentoring, coaching and 360° feedback.

A process, which is suited to all career stages, is working in triads or triangles. Involving three people, the triad or triangle, come together to choose when, where and how to meet and learn; and what to learn and practice.

This can involve self-coaching, peer coaching, using the resources as a mentor/coach, team development, resources to build programs from and a whole system approach to tap into the collective intelligence of a community of learners.

More junior staff will benefit from spending time working with and learning from their managers. One example of this is called 'paired learning' which has been shown to have significant benefits to patients and leads to powerful personal learning. This approach is based on a buddy system which enable the trainee and the manager to work together to support and learn from each other and while doing so, gain experience of their colleagues expertise and insights into the others perspective (Klaber et al; 2011).

In this chapter we have identified a number of generic developmental approaches that educationalists at any level might use in helping learners to acquire leadership competence, or indeed specific to using the CLCF.

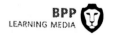

However, one aspect that is clear in the successful use of the CLCF to support enhanced leadership capacity across the NHS is the clinical role of tutors and trainees. If colleagues in these roles can familiarise themselves with the content of the CLCF, and then use it regularly and in an integrated way with acquisition of clinical skills then trainees will come to see leadership as just part and parcel of their everyday role.

Chapter summary

In this chapter we learned:

- It is important that leadership learning is incorporated within the mainstream curriculum, rather than regarded as something additional or even peripheral to that core.

- Insight gained through feedback or self assessment is vitally important to leadership development.

- Feedback and assessment tools help individuals identify where their leadership strengths and development needs lie.

- Dynamic learning methods such as action learning sets, paired learning and triads offer excellent environments for clinicians as part of workplace based leadership development.

- There is an excellent e-learning resource available on the National Learning Management System called LeAD which is appropriate for all clinical staff regardless of profession, specialty, or stage of training and offers one component of an overall leadership training and development programme.

Chapter references

Klaber B, Lee J, Abraham R, Smith L, Lemer C (2012). Paired Learning. A peer learning leadership development initiative for managers and clinicians in the NHS. London: Imperial College Healthcare NHS Trust.

King J (1999) Giving feedback. BMJ 318 (7200).

Spurgeon, P, and Klaber, R (2011) *Medical Leadership: A practical guide for tutors and trainees.* London: BPP Learning Media.

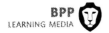

NHS Institute for Innovation and Improvement www.institute.nhs.uk/building_capability/general/lean_thinking.html

Revans R W (1978). *The ABC of action learning.* Birmingham: Wakelin.

Silverman JD, Jurtz SM, Draper J. (1990). *The Calgary-Cambridge approach to communication skills teaching, agenda led, outcome based analysis of the consultation.* Education in General Practice. 7 288–299.

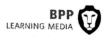

Appendix

Related and supporting reading

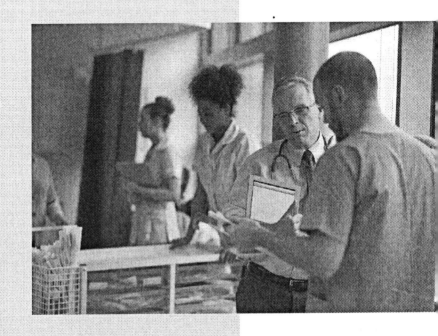

Related and supporting reading

British Association of Arts Therapists, *Suggestions from council on curriculum content*

British Dietetic Association (2008) *Curriculum framework for the pre-registration education and training of dieticians*

British and Irish Orthoptic Society (2008) *BIOS guidelines for implementing preceptorship*

British and Irish Orthoptic Society HNS KSF – *outline for Orthoptist Band 5*

British Psychological Society (2010) *Clinical Psychology Leadership Development Framework July 2010*

Charan R, S Drotter and J Noel (2001) *The Leadership Pipeline: How to Build the Leadership* Powered Company Chartered Society of Physiotherapy (2011) *CSP Physiotherapy Framework*

Chartered Society of Physiotherapy (2011) *CSP Learning & Development Principles*

College of Occupational Therapists (2006) *Post Qualifying Framework: A resource for occupational therapists* College of Occupational Therapists (2009 revised edition) *The College of Occupational Therapists' Curriculum Guidance for Pre-Registration Education*

College of Operating Department Practitioners (2009) *BSc in Operating Department Practice* Curriculum Document College of Optometrists (2009) *Scheme for Registration Trainee Handbook 2009*

College of Optometrists (2009) *Assessment Framework Optometrists*

College of Paramedics (2008) *Paramedic Curriculum Guidance and Competence Framework, 2nd edition*

Committee of Postgraduate Dental Deans and Directors (2006) *A curriculum for UK Dental Foundation Programme Training*

College of Podiatrists and the Society of Chiropodists and Podiatrists (2008) *Regulations and guidance for the accreditation of pre-registration education programmes in Podiatry leading to eligibility for membership of The Society of Chiropodists and Podiatrists Handbook, Edition 2*

Department of Health (2010) *The NHS Knowledge and Skills Framework (NHS KSF) and the Development Review Process*

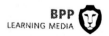

Department of Health (2008) *High Quality Care for All: NHS Next Stage Review Final Report*

Department of Health (2010) *Equity and excellence: Liberating the NHS* (White Paper)

Department of Health (2009) *Transforming Community Services: Enabling new patterns of provision*

Department of Health (2010) *Modernising Scientific Careers: The UK Way Forward*

Department of Health (2010) *Planning and Developing the NHS Workforce: The National Framework* Department of Health (2010) *Building a Safe and Confident Future: Implementing the recommendations of the Social Work Task Force*

Department of Health (2010) *Pharmacy in England: Building On Strengths – Delivering the Future* (White Paper)

Department of Health (2008) *Modernising allied health professions (AHP) careers: a competence-based career framework*

Department of Health (2010) *Preceptorship Framework for newly registered nurses, midwives and allied health professionals*

General Dental Council (2010) *Outcomes for registration*

General Medical Council (2009) *Tomorrow's Doctors: Outcomes and standards for undergraduate medical education*

Gitsham, M (2009) *Developing the Global Leaders of Tomorrow.* Ashridge Business School and the European Academy of Business in Society

Gronn P (2008) *The Future of Distributed Leadership, Journal of Educational Administration, 46(2), 141–58*

Hartley J and Bennington J (2010) *Leadership for Healthcare.* Policy Press: Bristol

Health Professions Council (2009) *Standards of education and training*

Health Professions Council (Various) *Standards of Proficiency*

Health Professions Council (2008) *Standards of conduct, performance and ethics*

Health Professions Council (2005) *Standards for Continuing Professional Development July 2005*

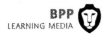

Heifetz R and Laurie D (2009) *Review: The work of Leadership by Heifetz and Laurie.* The Welsh NHS Confederation

Midwifery 2010 Midwifery 2020 – Delivering Expectations

MMC Inquiry (2008) *Aspiring to Excellence: Final Report of the Independent Enquiry into Modernising Medical Careers*

Mott MacDonald (2010) *Literature Review: Leadership Frameworks. Mott MacDonald: Bolton*

National Skills Academy Social Care (2009) *Leadership and management prospectus*

National Skills Academy Social Care (2010) *Overview and Key Messages May 2010*

NHS Institute for Innovation and Improvement and Academy of Medical Royal Colleges (2010) *Medical Leadership Competency Framework, 3rd edition*

NHS Institute for Innovation and Improvement (2006) *NHS Leadership Qualities Framework*

NHS Scotland (2009) Delivering Quality Through Leadership: NHS Scotland Leadership Development Strategy Nursing and Midwifery Council (2010) Standards for pre-registration nursing education: draft for consultation Royal College of Speech and Language Therapists (2007) Speech and Language Therapy Competency Framework to Guide Transition to Full RCSLT Membership

Royal College of Speech and Language Therapists CPD Framework – Human and Financial Leadership and Resource Management

Skills for Care and Development (2009) *Health and Social Care – National Occupational Standards*

Skills for Health, Shape a quality nursing workforce

Society and College of Radiographers (2007) *Learning and development framework for clinical imaging and oncology*

Society and College of Radiographers (2010) *Education and professional development strategy: new directions*

Society and College of Radiographers (2005) *A framework for professional leadership in clinical imaging and radiotherapy and oncology services*

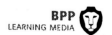

Spurgeon, P, Clark. J, and Ham C (2011) *Medical Leadership: From the dark side to centre stage,* Oxford Radcliffe Press: Oxford

Stanton E, Lemer C and Mountford J (eds) (2010) *Clinical Leadership: Bridging the divide.* Quay Books: London

Tamkin P, Pearson G, Hirsh W and Constable S (2010) *Exceeding Expectation: the principles of outstanding leadership.* The Work Foundation

Wilson A, Lenssen G, and Hind P (2007) *Leadership Qualities and Management Competencies for Corporate Responsibility. Ashridge Business School and the European Academy of Business in Society*

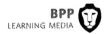

Appendix

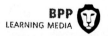

More titles in the Progressing your Medical Career Series

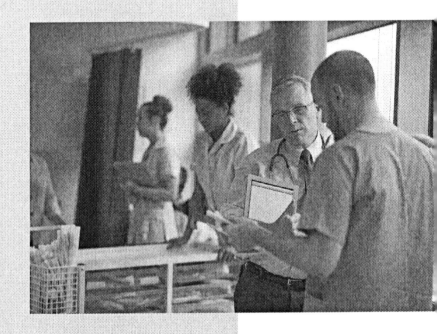

More titles in the Progressing your Medical Career Series

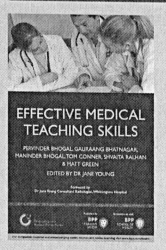

EFFECTIVE MEDICAL TEACHING SKILLS

PERVINDER BHOGAL, GAURAANG BHATNAGAR, MANINDER BHOGAL, TOM CONNER, SHVAITA RALHAN & MATT GREEN

EDITED BY DR JANE YOUNG

Foreword by
Dr Jane Young Consultant Radiologist, Whittington Hospital

£19.99
October 2011
Paperback
978-1-445379-55-5

We can all remember a teacher that inspired us, encouraged us and helped us to excel. But what is it that makes a good teacher and are these skills that can be learned and improved?

As doctors and healthcare professionals we are all expected to teach, to a greater or lesser degree, and this carries a great deal of responsibility. We are helping to develop the next generation and it is essential to pass on the knowledge that we have gained during our experience to date.

This book aims to cover the fundamentals of medical education. It has been designed to be a guide for the budding teacher with practical advice, hints, tips and essential points of reflection designed to encourage the reader to think about what they are doing at each step.

By taking the time to read through this book and completing the exercises contained within it you should:

- Understand the needs of the learner

- Understand the skills required to be an effective teacher

- Understand the various different teaching scenarios, from lectures to problem based teaching, and how to use them effectively

- Understand the importance and sources of feedback

- Be aware of assessment techniques, appraisal and revalidation

This book aims to provide you with a foundation in medical education upon which you can build the skills and attributes to become a competent and skilled teacher.

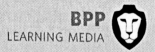

BPP LEARNING MEDIA

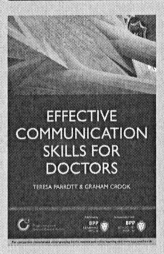
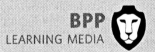

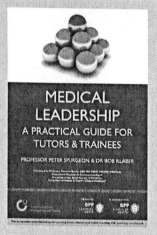
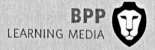

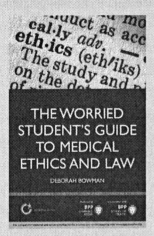
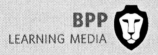

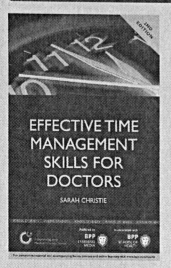
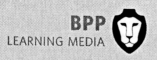

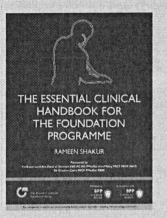
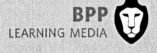

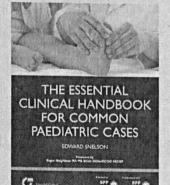
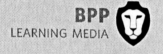